PRAISE FOR
THE CORE CONCEPTS OF MINDFUL EATING: PROFESSIONAL EDITION

Megrette Fletcher, in writing Core Concepts of Mindful Eating, has pointed us toward a different relationship with issues that are, for many of us, as enduring as they are painful. The idea that we can create a health promoting, enjoyable, balanced relationship with the food we eat without demeaning, criticizing, or feeling disgust toward, ourselves is hard to grasp. Yet in Core Concepts of Mindful Eating Megrette describes an array of techniques and perspectives that could, if embraced, lead to just such a change. She doesn't offer quick or easy answers, but does propose a way of considering the questions involved with establishing a positive relationship with our nutrition that can provide immediate sense of relief and excitement about the possibilities. — JOHN E. BRELSFORD PHD, LMHC

"*An ambitious book from a master teacher of mindful eating chock-full of valuable resources and exercises. What makes this book invaluable is Megrette's open-ended invitation to cultivate a nonjudgmental attitude both toward clients and toward oneself.*" – JEAN FAIN, HARVARD MEDICAL SCHOOL-AFFILIATED PSYCHOTHERAPIST AND AUTHOR OF "THE SELF-COMPASSION DIET"

OBTAIN CPE FROM SKELLY SKILLS FOR READING THIS BOOK!

Did you know that The Core Concepts of Mindful Eating also has a self-paced CPEU program? This program is accredited by The Commission of Dietetic Registration, CDR and is approved for 32 CPE by Skelly Skills.

Enjoy this self-paced program that includes:

- The Core Concepts of Mindful Eating ebook
- Detailed self-study guide and CPE exam.

Visit Skelly Skills to learn more about this program!

YOU CAN ALSO ACCELERATE YOUR LEARNING BY TAKING MEGRETTE'S LIVE TRAINING PROGRAM.

The program is an internet based, 10-week training. Each week you will enjoy working in a small group of 8 students to dive deep into the ideas, questions and practical application of mindful eating.

The live training program is offered three times a year: In the Winter - starting in January, Spring - starting in March and Fall - starting in September. This program is accredited by The Commission of Dietetic Registration, CDR and is approved for 40 CPEU for Registered Dietitians and Diet Technicians by Skelly Skills.

This program provides 20 live/20 self-study CPEU.

You will receive:

- 20-hours of live instruction, 10 session, 2-hour in length
- The Core Concepts of Mindful Eating book
- Guidance on meditation and a chance to lead a meditation
- Exposure to mindful eating assessment tools used in research
- Learning opportunities using your own clients and situations to advance your mindful eating skills and understanding

Visit megrette.com/training to learn more about this live training option.

PRAISE FOR THE CORE CONCEPTS OF MINDFUL EATING LIVE TRAINING

"Megrette has a gift for teaching mindful eating in a concise and practical manner. I enjoyed the Core Concepts in Mindful Eating course, as she presented the material with the perfect balance of her own professional experiences and the latest research, while keeping the client as the main focus." — LORI C.N. WELTER, MD, MS, MBA

"This was a comprehensive program encompassing learning that was both cognitive and experiential in the topics noted above. The program facilitator is an excellent teacher. She brings both a wealth of experience and learning tools to the course, and thoroughly models its principles. The program provided ample time for questions, participant interaction, feedback and support. As a result of this program, I feel very confident in my ability to teach these principles in both group and individual sessions. I am consistently using these concepts in my nutrition counseling. I conducted a lunchtime 'Introduction to Mindful Eating' program in my workplace and the participants asked for additional sessions. My own mindfulness practice has been enhanced by this program. I am very grateful for the opportunity to train with Megrette Fletcher, M.ED. RD CDE and to share this experience with a wonderful group of healthcare professionals." — BARBARA BOOTHBAY, MS RD

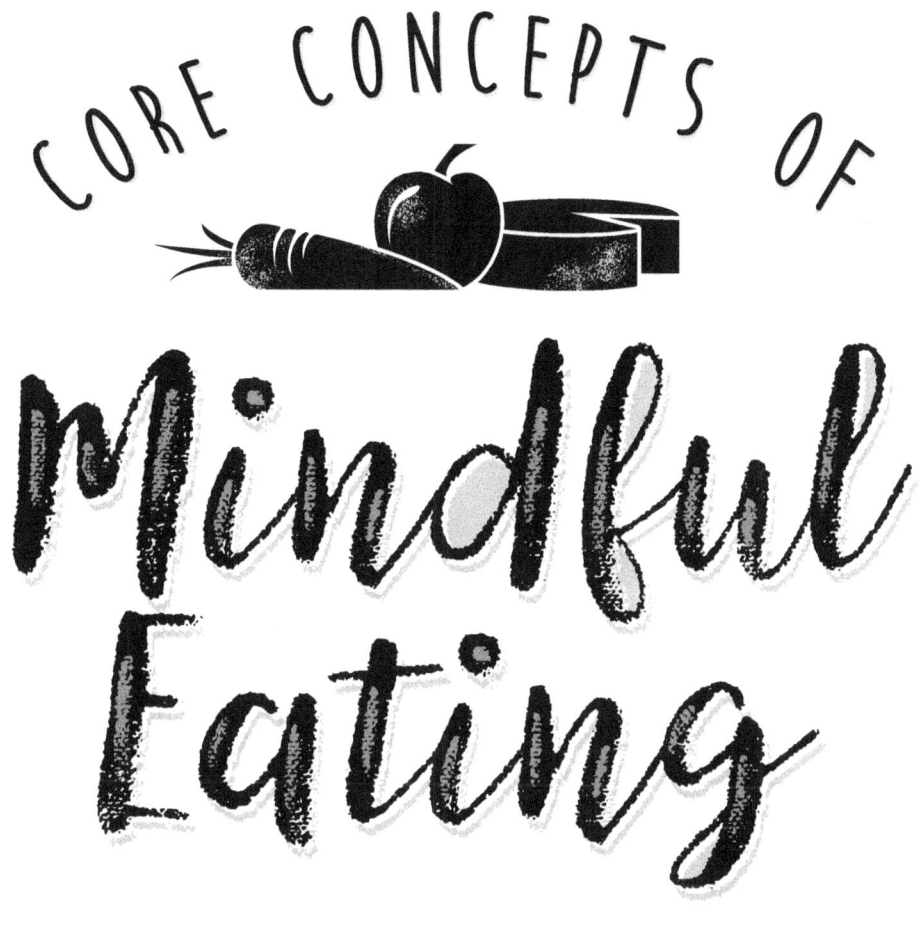

Core Concepts of Mindful Eating

The Professional Edition

By Megrette Fletcher M.Ed., RD CDE

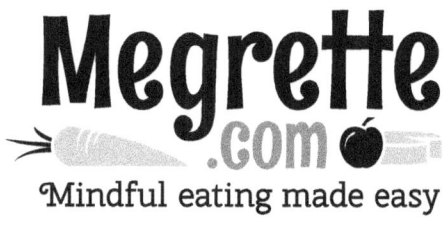

Mindful eating made easy

EPPING NH USA

©2017 by Megrette Fletcher
Megrette.com
80 Camp Lee Road
Epping NH 03042 USA
www.megrette.com

Cover design and illustrations: David Gillis
Illustrations: Sarah Fletcher
Copyediting: Sue Weston
All Rights Reserved.

ISBN: 978-0-692-85208-8

1. Mindful Eating 2. Nutrition

DEDICATION PAGE

This book is dedicated to:

My sister Sarah for her lifelong friendship.

Dh Amala for her nourishing spiritual friendship.

Sheila for her inspiring business friendship.

A portion of the sales of this book will be donated to support nonprofits mentioned:

The Center for Mindful Eating

The Center for Nonviolent Communication

The Health Education & Training Institute

The Center for Contemplative Mind in Society

The Association for Size Diversity and Health.

Table of Contents

Introduction
Why Mindful Eating? 6

A Reese's Peanut Butter Cup? 6
What Drives Your Decisions 7

SECTION ONE
The Spirit of Nonjudgment, Understanding Meditation & Defining Self-Kindness 12

    Introduction to Section One 13

Empathizing — David 14

Chapter 1
The Spirit of Nonjudgment 15
    The Unspoken Challenge of Nonjudgment 15
        Counseling Activity — Nonjudgment 16
        Going Deeper
        Debriefing the activity 16
    The Spirit of Motivational Interviewing (MI) 17
    Judgment and Shame: Conjoined Feelings 18
        Counseling Activity — What is Shame? 19
        Going Deeper
        Debriefing Shame 19
    Moving Past Shame: How Mindfulness Can Help 20
        Counseling Activity — Make Your Own Principles of Mindful Eating 21
        Going Deeper
        Debriefing the activity 21
        Counseling Activity — Thought Compass 22
        Going Deeper
        Debriefing a Thought Compass 23
    Chapter Summary
    The Spirit of Nonjudgment 25

Empathizing — Sita 26

Chapter 2
Meditation 27
    What Can Meditation Do for You? 28
    Reflecting 28
    What is mindfulness? 29
    Four Types of Mindfulness Meditations 32

    A3D Breathing Space 32
    Mindful Awareness in Three Stages 33
    Kindness and Compassion Meditation 34
    Traditional Metta Bhavna Meditation 35
    Meditations Script 36
        Counseling Activity 38
        Going Deeper
        Debriefing a meditation 38
    Counseling a debriefing session with clients or in a group 38
    Using a MI technique to debrief your counseling activities 39
    Returning to the first section of this chapter: Empathizing. 40
        Counseling Activity — Thought Compass 40
    Chapter Summary
    Meditation 41

Empathizing — Linda 42

Chapter 3
Defining Self-Kindness 43
    Reflecting 44
        Counseling Activity — Self-Kindness = Equal 45
        Going Deeper
        Debriefing Self-Kindness Activity 45
        Counseling Activity: Defining Self-Kindness 46
    Self-Kindness is a mental concept and an emotional experience. 46
    How to make the 13-inch journey 46
    Reflecting self-kindness for your clients 48
        Counseling Activity — Practicing Reflection 48
        Going Deeper
        Debriefing Practicing Reflection Statements 49

Counseling Options Using Motivational Interviewing to Explore Mindful Eating 49

Listening for Change Talk 50

    Counseling Activity — DARN 50

    Going Deeper
Debriefing Listening for Change Talk 50

    Counseling Activity — Shifting to Action Taken . 51

Keeping the Desire to Change Going 51

    Counseling Activity — Becoming All EARS 51

    Going Deeper
Debriefing Shifting to Action Activities 52

Softening Harsh Self-Talk 53

Merit 53

Counseling Tip 53

Setting the Intention 54

Seeing Barriers to Change 55

How does a client feel self-kindness? 55

Empathizing Revisited 55

Self-Compassion Self-Assessment 55

    Counseling Activity — Thought Compass 57

Chapter Summary
Defining Self-Kindness 58

SECTION TWO
Sensory/physical, Cognitive/thought, and Emotion/feelings 60

Introduction to
Section Two 61

The Mindful Eating Map 62

Empathizing — Sita 64

Chapter 4
Sensory Experience While Eating 65

Reflecting — Exploring Sensory Experience 65

    Counseling Activity — The Food Hook 66

Empathizing: Sensory Experience 67

    Counseling Activity — Thought Compass on
Sensory Experience 68

What is physical hunger? 68

    Counseling Activity — Hunger and Fullness 70

Six Phases of Eating 71

Understanding the Six Phases 71

    Going Deeper
Balancing Sensory Information with Self-Kindness . 72

Beckoning or Humming 73

    Counseling Activity — Try Beckoning or
Humming 73

Listening for Change Talk 73

    Counseling Activity — Discover, Explore, Play,
and Challenge 74

    Going Deeper
Debriefing Desire 74

DARN (Revisited) — Motivational
Interviewing Mnemonic for Hearing Change Talk ... 75

Chapter Summary
Sensory Experience While Eating 76

Empathizing — Sita 77

Chapter 5
Thought Experience 78

The Problem With Thoughts 78

Why Observe Your Thoughts? 79

The Benefit of Observation 79

    Counseling Activity — The Playbill 80

    Going Deeper
Debriefing The Playbill Activity 80

    Counseling Activity — Countering Thought
Stories 81

    Going Deeper
Debriefing Countering Stories Activity 81

How Mindfulness Can Help 81

The Time Machine 82

    Counseling Activity — Becoming an Observer .. 82

    Going Deeper
*Debriefing the Observing Thoughts
and Emotions Activity* 83

Creating Space for Your Thoughts 83

Turn Off the Monkey Mind When Eating 83

Permission, Freedom, and Space
The Solution for Restriction 84

    Counseling Activity — Evaluating Thoughts 84

  Thought Habits and Therapy 85

    Going Deeper
    Debriefing Evaluating Thoughts Activity 85

    Counseling Activity — Thought Compass on
    Thought Experience 85

  Chapter Summary
  Thought Experience 86

Empathizing — Linda 87

Chapter 6
Emotional Experience 88

  How Sensory and Emotional Experiences Are
  Similar 88

    Counseling Activity — Where Your Emotions
    are Felt 89

    Not All Experiences Are Pleasant 90

    Tolerating vs. Enjoying 90

    Counseling Activity — Evaluating Your Feelings 90

    Going Deeper
    Debriefing Evaluating Your Feelings Activity 91

  The Funny Thing About Feelings 91

    Counseling Activity — Feeling Your Feelings ... 92

    Going Deeper
    Debriefing the Feeling Your Feelings Activity 94

  Permission Is Surprisingly Powerful 94

  The Space for Your Feelings 94

  Creating Conditions for Acceptance 96

    Counseling Activity — Using the Mindful
    Eating Map 98

    Going Deeper
    Debriefing Using the Mindful Eating Map
    Activity 100

  How Your Gut Gets in the Way 100

    Counseling Activity — Gas, Brake, or Both? ... 100

    Going Deeper
    Debriefing Feeling Stuck 101

    Counseling Activity – Thought Compass
    Emotions 101

  Chapter Summary
  Emotional Experience 102

SECTION THREE
**Identifying Your Needs, Creating Your Intention, Advocating for Your Practice,
Teaching Your Passion** 103

  Introduction to
  Section Three 104

Empathizing — Jerome 105

Chapter 7
Identifying Your Needs 106

  Mindful Eating Map Step 3, Part One:
  Personal Needs 107

  Mental Wellness 107

    Counseling Activity — Healthy Mind Platter .. 108

    Going Deeper
    Debriefing the Healthy Mind Platter Activity 108

  Step 3, Part Two: Needs and Feelings 109

  Feelings as a Gateway to Your Needs 109

    Counseling Activity — Introduction to
    Nonviolent Communication 109

    Going Deeper
    Debriefing the List of Feelings Activity 111

  Needs, Feelings, and Counseling 111

    Counseling Activity — Exploring Feelings
    Using Complex Reflections 112

  Feeling Stuck 113

  Self-compassion, Feelings, and Needs 113

  Exploring Needs 113

    Counseling Activity — Meeting Your Needs 114

  Reducing Negative Experiences 115

    Going Deeper
    Debrief the Meeting Your Needs Activity 115

  Making Decisions to Meet Your Needs 115

  Using a Compassion Arrow 116

  Jerome's Compassion Arrow 116

    Going Deeper
    Debriefing the Compassion Arrow 117

    Counseling Activity — Thought Compass on
    Needs 117

  Chapter Summary
  Identifying Your Needs 118

Empathizing — David 119

Chapter 8
Creating Your Intention 120

- Why is positive energy more effective for a change? .. 120
- Reflecting 120
- Intention Helps You See Beyond the Quick Fix 120
- The Three Poisons 121
  - Counseling Activity — Creating Your Intention 122
  - *Going Deeper*
    Debriefing the Three Poisons 123
- How Is Intention Different From a Goal? 123
- How Does Intention Change Your Diet? 123
- Choosing Nutrition 124
- Sorting Out the Whys 124
  - Counseling Activity — "Nice Pants!" 125
  - *Going Deeper*
    Debriefing the "Nice Pants!" Activity 125
- Energy 126
- Body Function and Disease Prevention 126
- Why Nutrition Gets Confusing 127
- A Sense of Self-Care 127
  - Counseling Activity — Evaluating Effort 128
  - *Going Deeper*
    Debriefing Choices Activity 128
  - *Going Deeper*
    Debriefing Evaluating Effort Activity 128
- Tell a Friend 129
- Conclusion 129
  - Counseling Activity — Creating a Thought Compass of Creating Your Intention 129
- Chapter Summary
  Creating Your Intention 130

Empathizing — Linda 131

Chapter 9
Advocating for
Your Practice 132

Carnegie Hall 132
  Counseling Activity — Using the Practice Planning Worksheet 132
Section 1
What to Practice? 133
The Definition of Success 133
Section 2
Tracking Intention 134
Evaluate Your Results 135
  Going Deeper
  Debriefing the Practice Planning Worksheet Activity 135
Why Advocating Ethically? 136
Why Advocating Ethically is Personal 137
Enlightened Pizza? 137
The Memory of Food 138
Practice? Discipline? Diligence? 138
"Oops" 139
Renewing Your Mindful Eating Practice 139
  Counseling Activity — Thought Compass on Advocating for Your Practice 140
Chapter Summary
Advocating for Your Practice 141

Empathizing — Jerome 142

Chapter 10
Teaching Your Passion 143

Creating Engaged Learners 144
  Going Deeper
  Debriefing Engaged Learning 145
Make Learning Fun! 145
Where Do You Go From Here? 146
What You Have Learned! 147
Final Thoughts 149
Chapter Summary:
Teaching Your Passion 150

APPENDICES

A List of Needs 151
Practice Planning Worksheet 152
Hugs, Gratitude, and Thanks 153
Training Resources 154
Footnotes 155

Full Book Reviewers.

This book was reviewed by the following Mindful Eating, Motivational Interviewing, nutrition, and counseling experts to ensure that the information contained was accurate and effectively communicated the *Core Concepts of Mindful Eating*. This is an acknowledgement of and appreciation for their help, which enabled this book to be created.

Louise Adams, Master of Psychology (Clinical). Louise is a therapist, eating-disorder expert, meditation, self-compassion, and Health At Every Size expert, as well as the author of *Mindful Moments* (2016) and *The Non-Diet Approach Guidebook for Psychologists and Counsellors* (2014, with coauthor Fiona Willer, APD). When asked why mindful eating is important, she says, "Mindful Eating is empowering and peaceful, enjoyable and natural. Through Mindful Eating, many of my clients find their way out of disordered relationships with food and their body." You can learn more about Louise and her Mindful Eating, non-dieting work, which is based in Australia, at www.untrapped.me.

Elizabeth Berry, MS, RDN. Liz is a dietitian who is an expert in Mindful Eating, Motivational Interviewing, counseling, self-compassion, Nonviolent Communication, and meditation. When asked why mindful eating is important, she explains, "My mission is to communicate the joy of mindfulness in life and with food and the entire eating experience. There is far too much judgment and shame around food choices, amounts, and body types." You can learn more about Liz and her amazing work at www.berrynutrition.com.

Mary Saucier Choate, M.S., R.D.N., L.D. Mary is a dietitian with expertise in Health At Every Size. When asked why mindful eating is important, she says, "My own experience has proven it to be a compassionate self-care process."

Sondra Gudmundson, MS, RD, LD, CDE. Sondra is a dietitian and Mindful Eating teacher. She holds expertise in Mindfulness, Motivational Interviewing, and counseling and has intentional practice with meditation and self-compassion. When asked why mindful eating is important, she says, "Mindful eating is a safe, connecting, and satisfying activity that nurtures one's body and also spirit. When practiced regularly, mindfulness with eating serves as an internal compass of how we can approach other situations in life with a similar manner of awareness and nonjudgment. Mindful Eating is truly kindness to oneself."

Maryann Jacobsen, MS, RD. Maryann is a dietitian and the author of Fearless Feeding and *How to Raise a Mindful Eater*. When asked why mindful eating is important, she explains, "I believe it's an important — and missing — component of teaching people of all ages to live a healthy lifestyle. Too many people are not aware of what Mindful Eating is and the benefits it can bring to their life." You can learn more about Maryann at www.MaryannJacobsen.com

Cheryl Wasserman, M.A., L.P.C., N.C.C. Cheryl is a therapist and former board member of The Center for Mindful Eating. When asked why mindful eating is important, she says, "Mindful Eating has changed my life in that it has taught me to slow down, be lovingly present with myself, as I savor every aspect of whatever is before me." You can learn more about Cheryl and her work at www.mindfuleatingforlife.com.

Lori C.N. Welter, MD, MS, MBA. Lori is a physician specializing in physiatry, including spine and sports medicine, and cognitive disorders and brain-injury treatment. She has additional expertise in eating disorders, Mindfulness-based practices, and meditation. In her presentations, she illustrates the concept of Mindful Eating with a wicked sense of humor supported by the latest, greatest research. When asked why mindful eating is important, she says, "It restores our freedom. Listen carefully, and you can almost hear what your body is telling you. Be mindful, and you will make your food choices not with guilt or shame, but with loving kindness and a healthy appreciation of what your body needs." Learn more about Dr. Welter and her practice at MyMindfulMD.com and DrLoriWelter.com.

"Food is one of the greatest pleasures of life, and pleasure is good medicine."

— Marsha Hudnall, MS RD, President of Green Mountain at Fox Run

INTRODUCTION

Why Mindful Eating?

The question Why? is central to the concept of Mindful Eating. For example, why choose Mindful Eating to address longstanding, typically challenging nutrition and eating concerns? What is it about Mindful Eating that has piqued your interest? What are you really looking for?

A Reese's Peanut Butter Cup?

At first glance, it appears that there are a lot of options when it comes to recommending a food or eating plan. Yet, if you look at these options, they can be divided into two categories.

One category is dieting that encourages the individual to restrict his or her intake of food. This includes the typical calorie-restricted diet, such as eating 1,200 calories a day. There has been a wave of information indicating that these simple calorie-restrictive diets don't work. The billion-dollar industry that surrounds weight loss, and savvy corporations that sell "diets," a.k.a. restrictive eating, have changed their marketing strategies. It's no longer as easy to spot a "diet" as it was in the past.[1, 2]

Disguising restrictive eating has become very clever, and examples of how this hidden restriction appears include: eating a specific type of food that is defined as "Paleo," "clean," "ketogenic" or "raw"; or restricting when you eat, for example not eating meat or dairy before 6 P.M., or not eating after 7 P.M., or eating five small meals a day. These plans and programs may be nutritionally adequate, but emotionally and psychologically, they are lacking.

The other category is not dieting at all. You choose to stop focusing on appearance and weight-loss outcomes and, instead, focus on your direct experience and begin understanding your behavioral patterns. This concept is mindfulness.

When you combine mindfulness with eating, you have Mindful Eating. This suggestion, at first, feels shocking and counterintuitive. Many professionals have a sense of urgency to do *something*, especially with the rising rates of obesity, heart disease, and diabetes. Even the mere suggestion of not dieting challenges the ethics of health care. This underlying discomfort with the idea of a non-restrictive-eating plan has opened the marketing door to what appears to be a new option, the non-restrictive-eating weight-loss diet. Could this be the Reese's Peanut Butter Cup that dietitians have all been craving? Could the non-restrictive-eating weight-loss diet, an amazing combination, become the all-around best-sounding option ever?

Unfortunately, a few bites into a non-restrictive-eating weight-loss diet will leave an empty taste in your mouth. The conflicting concept of a non-restrictive-eating plan designed to promote weight loss is a Trojan horse. It may seem like a gift, but if the plan focuses on weight loss, this gift horse carries the destructive enemy of restrictive eating, which will sabotage motivation. Regardless of what they're called, programs, plans, or diets that focus on appearance, including weight loss, are restrictive by nature. Knowing what to do is even harder now, because dietitians and health-care providers are having trouble identifying restrictive-eating plans from non-restrictive-eating plans.

WHAT DRIVES YOUR DECISIONS

For the last 100 years, dieting has grown into a multi-billion-dollar industry. Scientists, researchers, governments, and health-care providers are questioning whether specific calorie- or nutrient-focused diets even work. This questioning comes from the logical suspicion that if dieting worked, wouldn't everyone be thin? Instead, as a nation, and in the world, people are getting bigger. In 2013, obesity became classified by the American Medical Association as a chronic illness. This change in classifying obesity as an illness was made with the hope of bringing more services, tools, and support to individuals who wish to lose weight. However, many body-acceptance advocates objected to this change in classification, stating that defining obesity as a chronic illness pathologizes the individual and does not recognize the inherent flaws associated with the Body Mass Index tool, and ultimately only benefits a size-focused weight-loss industry.

Having a BMI greater than normal weight does not mean that you are unhealthy, or indicate the presence of illness, just as having a normal weight does not mean you are healthy or indicate the absence of illness. Determining health is not as simple as stepping on a scale. Health cannot be thought of as a "one-size-fits-all" state, but instead is best described as an ever-changing, complex state that balances the physical, emotional, and psychological needs of the individual. As a society, we are waking up to the reality that a simple solution like "dieting" can't possibly address the biological, psychological, societal, cultural, and environmental factors of a person.

Could eating with awareness be the solution to the biological, psychological, societal, cultural, and environmental challenges an individual faces regarding food and eating? It might be, it might not. Long-term studies are still needed to prove that mindful eating is effective.[3] If there isn't overwhelming evidence to support Mindful Eating, why should I consider learning about it? Mindful Eating can't offer guarantees or promises about weight loss, because Mindful Eating isn't about size, shape, or outward appearance. Mindful Eating is about training your mind to become aware of options and choices. You can see that this is the opposite of dieting, which is teaching you to limit options and restrict choices.

The lovely part of Mindful Eating is that, when you practice a new skill, it gets easier. As you develop the skill of awareness, you are better able to see choices, options, and solutions to the biological, psychological, societal, cultural, and environmental factors that are not supporting you. Unlike dieting and restrictive eating, Mindful Eating does not promote psychological, emotional, or physical problems. In fact, research has identified that Mindful Eating helps[ibid]:

- Decrease portions
- Decrease food cravings
- Decrease emotional eating
- Decrease binge-eating behavior
- Decrease depression and anxiety
- Decrease emotional stress
- Decrease automatic or habitual behavioral response to food.
- Improve food selection
- Increase a sense of autonomy and control surrounding food and eating choices.
- Improve body image
- Improve stress management

The greatest benefit of Mindful Eating — that it does not cause harm – is woefully underreported. In fact, the evidence shows that Mindful Eating actually heals the psychological, emotional, or physical harm caused by restrictive eating.

MEME TELLS HER STORY

My journey in Mindful Eating has been a slow but steady one. I found Mindful Eating when it felt almost unbearable to spend any more brain power worrying about my food and lifestyle choices, constantly concerned that I was not a good dietitian if I wasn't skinny and always eating "healthy" food. I'd heard about this way of eating and thought it surely wouldn't work for me, but I might as well try it.

I'd spent so many years resisting my hunger cues and cravings; I always saw those as signs that I was doing something wrong. Am I not eating enough protein? Did I have too much sugar today? I should be eating more vegetables?

It was a constant battle between my mind and my body, and it was growing increasingly unpleasant. On top of that, my self-confidence and body image were ever plummeting, and I felt that my worth was tied to my weight and my diet. I was either thinking about what I should be eating, what I could eat, how much I needed to workout that day, or feeling guilty because of the choices I had made.

Mindful Eating has given me so much more than being free from the diet-shame spiral. It has given me the confidence to trust my body and intuition. I no longer spend countless hours calculating calories or beating myself up when I eat something not deemed as healthy. I make choices based on my hunger level and what my body needs at that moment. I no longer feel the need to have cheat meals or last suppers; that food will always be there if I crave it. I no longer eat food just for its health benefits; instead, I eat food because it gives me energy, nourishes my body, and/or tastes delicious. I respect my body by making the right choices for me at that moment.

There are times when I make decisions based on my old way of thinking, but now I am able to see those moments through a curious and compassionate lens and use them as teachable moments for both myself and my clients. Mindful Eating isn't always easy, but it is more than worth it!

HOW MINDFUL EATING HELPS

Mindful Eating teaches you how to become aware of choice surrounding food and eating. Practicing Mindful Eating is choosing to strengthen the new skill of awareness. With practice, a person's ability to see and discover more choices and options increases. When clients begin to see new choices, there is a shift in their energy. They are filled with "whys" designed to explore possibilities and options that are present. Mindfulness and Mindful Eating can also help you sit with challenging feelings such as anger, frustration, sadness, confusion, doubt, and uncertainty without reacting or having to feed the feeling. When you commit to a Mindful Eating practice, you are choosing to learn how to pay attention, on purpose. In time, with practice, the skill of awareness becomes strong, and the natural curiosity of mindfulness becomes second nature. You can see and experience the benefit from a committed Mindful Eating practice in every moment because you can identify more options and can enjoy the spectrum of choices. Food and eating is no longer limited to the binary option of "eat this/don't eat that!" There is room in every food choice for enjoyment, enthusiasm, and fun!

This ability to recognize choice is enhanced by learning to move away from judgment, to observe each choice nonjudgmentally. The removal of "should," "must," or "have to" from the equation opens you up to a world of options. This nonjudgmental aspect of mindfulness allows you to explore all choices equally without reacting to cravings or fears. Developing the ability to observe and "be with" without reacting to thoughts, physical sensations, and fears increases choice because it moves a person away from his/her habitual patterns. The ability to hold a ***curious stance***[4] seems to remove previous obstacles, again allowing more choice.

An additional benefit of mindfulness and Mindful Eating is emerging evidence that mindfulness strengthens synaptic connections and creates new thought patterns.[5, 6] These physical changes to the brain may be why, over time, mindfulness and Mindful Eating become easier and are associated with improved mood, contributing to an overall improved sense of well-being.[7]

LINN TELLS HER STORY:

Why mindfulness and Mindful Eating? Because it can change your life and bring you back to who you truly are. I feel like my own story has finally come full circle, through challenges with food, eating, and body image, back to a healthy healing relationship with same. And eventually this journey gave me heartfelt passion, new direction, and a new career.

I grew up eating healthy, home-cooked meals made by my health-conscious mum, yet I spent most of my late teens and early twenties battling my body, my weight, and my relationship with food. I was that emotional eater, the one who would drown her sorrows with ice cream or a big bag of sweets … I got trapped in a vicious cycle of sugary food cravings, poor food choices, energy spikes, followed by crashes, then back to more cravings.

Looking back at my eating story, connecting the dots, what started out as a sweet tooth spiraled into 10 years of disordered eating after being called fat in my late teens. I spent a few years starving myself, which only exacerbated my sugar cravings, driven by my low blood sugars. This was of course not a sustainable way to keep my weight under control. It eventually went back on and some. I was miserable with my body and I used food to make myself feel better…

I had for a long time what I now call "a dieting mindset." You know, you're on a diet, it starts on a Monday and you are "being good." This moralizing of food had to stop … So rather than cutting any particular foods out, I worked on cutting the guilt out.

Using a mindful approach of nonjudging, alongside re-learning to listen to my hunger and satiety cues, was my major pivot point in healing my relationship with food and eating. I went on to study Nutritional Therapy, the science of food and health and how the two are deeply intertwined. I've been working as a Nutritional Therapist in private practice since I graduated.

Through mindfulness we create awareness, we learn to listen in. Then we can let go of numbers, of the scales, of the counting. And we reconnect with our own inner wisdom. For me it's been a process of opening up to making NOURISHING choices based on self-care compassion. I've changed my way of looking at cooking and eating, from a chore to a way of being CREATIVE, artistic, and having FUN! To caring and sharing. From all this constant unfolding of change has come new opportunities; more health, better emotional expression, and deeper fulfillment.

I plant, I grow, I cook, I eat. I create. I love. I am. Food & Eating has been part of my path of personal growth — a colourful road to Whole Self Health. And you can have it, too.

GETTING REAL, GETTING HONEST

As wonderful as becoming aware is, it is easy to become distracted when you eat. This is the reason self-compassion is one of the roots of Mindful Eating. When you practice Mindful Eating, you attempt to drop into the present moment and stay there, regardless of what arises. You compassionately acknowledge the typical distractions that can pull you from the present moment. These distractions can range from smelling food, feeling happy, to gaining new insights. One of the biggest distractions is the thought, wish, or belief that Mindful Eating connects you with only happy moments and that it always feels great. This is considered a distraction because eating mindfully won't magically make your life wonderful. If you believe that Mindful Eating will make your life or food choices perfect, you will become distracted by an endless amount of disappointment when this doesn't happen. Life is a mixed bag of emotions that include the dark and the light thoughts and all the stuff in between. Mindful Eating is being with your life, as it is right now, not just the parts of life you like! As Jon Kabat-Zinn says, "Mindfulness means paying attention in a particular way, on purpose, in the present moment, and nonjudgmentally."

The simplicity of mindfulness and Mindful Eating is a draw for many people. Yet, this simplicity can also bring some confusion.

MARSHA TELLS HER STORY:

As a registered dietitian nutritionist, my refuge was eating well from a nutritional standpoint. But when I discovered Mindful Eating, I realized that eating well encompassed a whole lot more than vitamins and minerals.

I discovered Mindful Eating before I knew that's what it was called. I joined Green Mountain at Fox Run in the mid-1980s. Thelma Wayler, RD, the founder of this pioneering nondiet retreat for women, understood that restriction such as you see with weight-loss diets frequently interferes with a person's ability to make supportive choices when it comes to eating. As dieting began to take over the American psyche, she founded Green Mountain to help women learn how to eat instead of starve. Central to that learning was developing trust in the ability to make decisions in your own best interest. As far as eating went, the program focused on helping women tune into their bodies and minds to decide what, when, and how much to eat. When we had Jon Kabat-Zinn as a guest speaker, we adopted the term "mindful eating."

Mindful Eating helped me find a nurturing relationship with food that supported my body, mind, and soul, and it helped me better help my clients find the same. As women who struggle with eating and weight — many of them having struggled for much of their lives — my clients are essentially lost when it comes to feeding themselves. All the conflicting advice they read or hear, as well as all the failure they experience trying to follow that advice, leaves them confused and chaotic around food. The most common reaction I hear when they learn about Mindful Eating is relief and hope.

For the last 30 years, I've had the privilege of sharing that discovery with the women who come to Green Mountain at Fox Run, a retreat founded to help women stop dieting and learn how to truly take care of themselves. Mindful Eating has always been at the core of our program because it represents a sustainable approach to eating that truly supports well-being. What could be better than that?

I've stayed committed to Mindful Eating because, based on both personal and professional experience, I believe it is the most sustainable approach to eating well. It allows for all the roles food plays in our lives, which includes enjoyment. There is plenty of research to back up my belief, but the most important fact is that I see how Mindful Eating changes the lives of the women with whom I work. Mindful Eating is foundation to true self-care, to help a person live a healthier, happier life focused on what is important to them, instead of being mired in struggles with eating and weight.

SO, HOW DO YOU START?

This book is written for health-care professionals, specifically dietitians, nutritionists, counselors, and health coaches, many of whom are new to the concept of Mindful Eating. For this reason, the book is written in first person. My hope is that this will allow you to experience Mindful Eating like a client. There are also concepts in the book that can expand your counseling skills. In these examples, I will refer to the dietitian specifically.

Throughout this book, you will meet four "friends," or patient profiles, that I will use to explore different counseling situations. Prior to each chapter, one of these four friends will help you understand how Mindful Eating is experienced and how it sounds in a counseling session.

These four friends will also join us as you make this journey. Our first destination is **Section One**, which will explore nonjudgment, meditation, and self-kindness. I call these the "Roots" of mindful eating.

Section Two will build on our learning of nonjudgment, meditation, and self-kindness and allow the mind to focus and remain present with sensory/physical, cognitive/thought, and emotional/feelings.

Section Three offers you a chance to teach the above six skills to your clients. You will develop tools and techniques to help you communicate the concept of Mindful Eating in ways that do not promote restrictive eating (a.k.a. dieting). How? By identifying your needs, creating your intention, advocating for your practice, and teaching your passion.

In Sections Two and Three, you will get to explore and use the Mindful Eating Map.

Each chapter will follow a five-part format:

Empathizing – This section will precede each chapter and will give you more information about the client that will be presented in the chapter.

Connecting — Funny stories or mistakes that may help connect and join these concepts together.

Counseling Activity – Techniques you may try, to explore your learning, to help you imagine a session with one of the four clients you will get to know throughout the book.

Going Deeper — You will have an opportunity to decide what was effective and what wasn't.

Chapter Summary – This will cover the following:
> *Hooray!* Review the counseling tools you just learned.
> *Oops!* Review struggles you might encounter.
> *Tada!* Review the action steps of the chapter.

Meet our four friends

These are the clients who will help us learn more about the Core Concepts of Mindful Eating.

LINDA is a middle-aged woman with a long history of trying new programs and diets to change some aspect of her health. She has verbalized a fear of "failing again" and feels an urgent need to change her diet and lose 30 pounds. As you meet Linda, listen for a deeper pattern of disordered eating behavior. Linda was recently diagnosed with prediabetes, and she was told to lose weight to cure this problem.

DAVID is a young man who is disabled after a motor-vehicle accident. He is in chronic pain, and walking and lifting objects are very difficult for him. David was trained in culinary arts and is a "foodie." He is underweight, and he would like to eat better, feel better, and regain the 14 pounds he has lost.

SITA is a college student who calls herself a vegetarian and sometimes vegan. She knows she is "overweight" and has expressed a desire to be healthier. She likes to say, "I love the way I look, but I don't really." She says, "I'm OK with my size," and is very clear that she is not interested in weight loss. She likes learning, she reads a lot on the internet, and she feels that, since she started college, her vegetarian diet hasn't been balanced, and this is her goal.

JEROME is a normal-weight, but very picky, 13-year-old who participates in a variety of sports. His mother, Myra, is a child-care provider who is struggling with her son and his eating habits, which are disruptive to the family. Jerome is at the session to improve the variety of his diet and to eat a healthier diet.

SECTION ONE

The Spirit of Nonjudgment, Understanding Meditation & Defining Self-Kindness

INTRODUCTION TO
Section One

In Section One, you will spend time learning about the three foundational concepts that underpin Mindfulness and Mindful Eating. These concepts I call "the roots of mindful eating" and they are: nonjudgmental observation, meditation, and self-kindness. Learning to apply these concepts in a counseling session is the purpose of Section Two and Three of this book. These terms will shift from a theoretical definition to a teachable concept that you can share with your clients. In time and with supportive practice, these concepts will become an effortless skill that offers you the dietitian an endless way to connect with your clients and yourself!

HOW SECTION ONE IS SET UP

In Chapter 1, you will learn about the spirit of nonjudgment and how nonjudgment is a foundational concept in Mindfulness, Mindful Eating, and motivational interviewing. In this chapter you will explore why a nonjudgmental stance is the best way to avoid shame, a toxic emotion that destroys motivation and erodes a counseling relationship. The chapter ends with learning a new skill called Thought Compass, which is a way to organize, understand, and make connection with new concepts.

Chapter 2 introduces you to meditation. Meditation will help you cultivate Mindfulness and allows you to explore your own mind. Meditation is intended as a way for you to practice the skill of nonjudgmental observation. If Mindful Eating is the direction you would like to move toward, Chapter 2 offers you two brief meditations for your counseling sessions. The chapter ends with creating a Thought Compass about meditation, asking you to organize your thoughts and knowledge and try to create some connections with your existing knowledge and the new concepts presented.

Chapter 3 explores the concept of self-kindness, which is one part of self-compassion. In Chapter 3, you will begin to see that even though the actual journey of change is only 13 inches long — the distance from your thoughts to your heart — moving information those few inches requires a surprisingly large amount of self-compassion, specifically self-kindness. In Chapter 3, you will have an opportunity to learn and use motivational interviewing to teach self-kindness. Chapter 3 explores the concept of merit, which can help you remain nonjudgmental and support your client throughout the change process. The chapter ends with creating a Thought Compass about self-kindness and self-compassion. In this space, take advantage of the opportunity to make your own 13-inch journey and connect your existing knowledge, experience, and personal understanding with the information presented.

EMPATHIZING - DAVID

"My background is in culinary arts. Once I got out of college, I decided to join the Marines. I served 5 years as a Marine chef. It was a great job because I used to cook for all the officers and officials, and I traveled to really interesting places like Japan and Hawaii. I loved my job but that ended after I was in a motor vehicle accident. I was the passenger in a car that was t-boned by a large truck. I have had so many surgeries to repair the right side of my body where the truck crushed me that I stopped keeping track. It seems that as a result of these injuries, I also have arthritis. I know that I am losing weight, and my doctor is concerned. We both agree I need to eat better."

— David

CHAPTER 1
The Spirit of Nonjudgment

"It is never too late to give up your prejudices."
— Henry David Thoreau

The concept of nonjudgment is a fundamental skill for effective counseling. Intellectually, the idea of nonjudgment appears straightforward. However, the moment you wake up and go about your daily business, you are likely to get lost in the rush and bustle of the day, and remaining nonjudgmental becomes much more challenging. In this chapter, you will explore the benefits of a nonjudgmental mindset, some ways to cultivate a nonjudgmental stance, and the science behind why nonjudgment is a foundational concept in Mindfulness, Mindful Eating, and motivational interviewing. Understanding nonjudgment and becoming more nonjudgmental will help your Mindful Eating journey, but even more interesting, I find, is that it will help you become a happier person.[8, 9, 10]

Sarah Roberts[11] explains, "Where acceptance and nonjudgment are concerned, acceptance may decrease stress by helping us let go of control and accept the facts." Roberts, a psychologist and the director of the MindSpace Clinic in Quebec, says, "Nonjudgment may make us happier by cutting out secondary emotions (e.g., getting angry because we're anxious; feeling guilty because we're depressed) and the stories we tell ourselves about certain experiences." Furthermore, "seeing unpleasant or difficult situations for exactly what they are — without getting wrapped up in our stories about the situations — allows us to use them as opportunities for growth." Roberts concludes, "Multiple (nonmutually exclusive) mechanisms have been proposed: greater appreciation of life via increased present-moment awareness; greater productivity as a result of improved attention; the joy and ease generated by acceptance and nonjudgment; and a decrease in the self-discrepancy gap."

THE UNSPOKEN CHALLENGE OF NONJUDGMENT

Can you think of some reasons you might unintentionally fall into a judgmental stance?

CONNECTING

For myself, it is being rushed and making faulty assumptions about my client's motivation for being at an appointment. I confess, I always assume they know why they are seeing a dietitian/diabetes educator. Dang it, after 25 years of counseling, I still forget that this isn't always the case.

COUNSELING ACTIVITY

When you are ready, pause and close your eyes, place the book in your lap and sit, feet flat on the ground and hands resting comfortably in your lap. Take a breath, then exhale, letting your breath slowly leave your body. During these few deep breaths, let go of any thoughts of what you are currently working on. These deep breaths will help you empathize — or begin to be "with" the problem that most of your clients are facing every day. The problem is judgment. Think for a moment and remember when you felt judged. You probably don't need to go too far into the past to remember an event. Chances are, it happened in the last hour.

Judgment can be small, David says.

People don't even have to say anything to me, just how they look at me. I can almost hear their thoughts wondering what's wrong with me. I walk like Frankenstein after an all-night bender, but I lack the facial scars and a cane, so there is nothing obvious-looking to tell people that I am injured.

Judgment can also be from the past.

That last dietitian I met was at rehab, but I got the feeling she didn't believe me. Like she thought I was lying when I told her I wasn't hungry.

COUNSELING ACTIVITY – **NONJUDGMENT**

Connect with the feeling that people are forming judgments and opinions about you. Can you describe the feeling? Would you label it Pleasant, Neutral, or Unpleasant?

Now, imagine a specific person you associate with this feeling of being judged. Imagine this person is going to teach you how to take care of yourself. This person is going to explain how to change your diet, eating, or activity.

Did feeling judged help you to learn, to become receptive to knowledge, to feel compassionate toward yourself? Or did this feeling have the opposite effect? Did it prevent you from learning, make feel you less receptive to knowledge, to close down your compassion for yourself and other people?

Now take a deep breath and ask yourself, What if the person who is judging you is yourself? Holding a nonjudgmental stance is all-inclusive — it includes yourself as well as other people. In the pages ahead, remember that the best way to teach Mindful Eating is to practice eating mindfully yourself. This practice includes nonjudgmental observation of yourself as much as it does your clients.

GOING DEEPER
Debriefing the activity

1. Take a moment and write down what you liked about connecting with the feeling of judgment.
2. Now list what you disliked about the activity.
3. What would you change after completing this activity? What areas of awareness were heightened?
4. Spend some time in reflection, asking yourself the following four questions:

- How have I observed the concept of nonjudgment be presented?
- How can I convey the concept of nonjudgment using my own words and experiences?
- Have I had an opportunity to teach this concept?
- How do I receive feedback about nonjudgment. When I receive feedback, how do I use this to change?

The Spirit of Motivational Interviewing (MI)

The concept of nonjudgment is complex and difficult to put in words and harder to put into practice. When I first started to use the Concepts of Mindful Eating with my clients, I realized that my counseling skills were not effective. I began searching for effective techniques and counseling training to facilitate a more nonjudgmental counseling approach. The most helpful approach for me was Motivational Interviewing, or MI. If you are not familiar with Motivational Interviewing, it is defined by William R. Miller and Stephen Rollnick, in their book *Motivational Interviewing: Helping People Change* (3rd edition)[12] as "a collaborative, goal-oriented style of communication with particular attention to the language of change. It is designed to strengthen personal motivation for and commitment to a specific goal by eliciting and exploring the person's own reasons for change within an atmosphere of acceptance and compassion."

This book will give you a taste of MI and it can help you effectively become more nonjudgmental, however it can not replace a live 2- or 3-day MI training. Think of this books as a primer or a way to explore MI if you are new or have forgotten any of the techniques. The first aspect of MI that you will explore is how to develop a client-centered approach. In MI, it simply begins with cultivating the spirit of MI.

MI identifies four qualities that define the "spirit" of each MI session. I have found that these four qualities also provide a great way for you to *move toward*[13] a more nonjudgmental stance.

- *Collaboration.* Counseling is a collaboration between two experts: the client/person and the counselor/helper. Beginning a session is described as an invitation to "dance." You are mentally asking yourself, "I would like this client to give me permission to move through the change process with them." You are not asking permission to start a wrestling match, where you fight with the client to accept your thoughts, opinions, and views. There are no power struggles because you avoid creating the impression that you have the answers. I know, the "But I do!" thought just flashed through your mind, and the compassionate wish to help someone is in your throat. Swallow. Breathe. This tiny moment of desire is what prompts us to offer unsolicited advice. Every counselor needs help and support to practice suppressing that compassionate Righting Reflex, which is the desire to help another person by telling them what to do. Of course, it's OK that this desire is present. Focus on becoming aware of and honest about your own values or agenda. Meditation is a great tool to help with this "awareness and honesty" business.

- *Acceptance.* Creating an absolute regard for the client is a great place to start. This regard can be described as an unconditional, positive, and nonjudgmental space that we hold for each client. The practice of unconditional acceptance is a challenge for all professionals and the reason Mindful Eating training includes a daily contemplative practice, such as mindfulness meditation. Among the benefits of mindfulness, consistent meditation promotes acceptance of ourselves and our own very real limitations.

- *Compassion.* This is the ability to be with another person's suffering. The skill to be with suffering in acceptance and collaboration is a challenge[14] and can be developed only with consistent practice. It is easy to forget that at the heart of compassion is the desire to work for the benefit of the client and not for yourself.

- *Evocation.* The term means to "call forth."[15] In regard to counseling, it is the ability to call forth the wisdom, experience, and expertise of the client's own change process. Imagine thinking before you start a session with your client, "My client is fully able to change and has no deficit nor is lacking anything to change." How might this thought shift your counseling energy?

It takes courage to bring this spirit into your counseling session. The benefit will likely be a counseling session that is filled with energy, that is more effective and less stressful. Why? To me, the answer is straightforward. Judgment is best used to evaluate tangible things such as labs, objects, and data. Judgment, however, is ineffective for subjective information, including behaviors, people, feelings, likes, dislikes, hopes, dreams, memories, and preferences. While I could not produce for a colleague a citation for this distinction about judgment, I would like to make an argument for my belief.

Subjective information is dynamic and influenced by many variables, and it is often associated with a person's self-view. For example, if you shared with someone that you liked the earthy taste of beet greens, and the other person reacted by saying, "Oh my GOSH! I hate those. You can't like them," you might be surprised by the intensity of response. This comment might hit even closer to home: If beet greens were a food that you associate with your culture — a food linked not just to your immediate family, but also to your extended family, friends, neighbors, or region — liking or disliking beet greens is not something that can be judged as "right/wrong" or "can/can't." It is a preference. When our choices and preferences are not accepted, something shifts in our relationships.

CONNECTING

I thought that I had solid counseling skills as a dietitian. I had always been interested in improving my counseling, as a way to be more effective, and I would pay to have supervision and take day long seminars. However, after twenty years I decided that I need to be better than "good". I choose to take a 3-day MI training. The training was amazing, and I was hooked. I thought that MI would be "easy" and that because I was "good" as counseling, that I would breeze through the coded evaluation process. That didn't happen. I received wonderful, detailed suggestions on how I could improve my counseling. The MI training process has improved my listening skills and that has helped me to be more effective at teaching mindful eating. It is essential that you have good counseling skills if you want Mindful Eating to be effective. If you are like me, and don't have a degree in counseling (and aren't planning on getting one) then consider committing to a live MI training.

JUDGMENT AND SHAME: CONJOINED FEELINGS

If a person experiences the feeling of being judged, shame will likely follow. What is shame? Brené Brown, PhD, defines shame as "the intensely painful feeling or experience that we are flawed and, therefore, unworthy of connection or belonging." I offer the following example to illustrate how shame can develop. This example shows the connection of judgment and shame.

Shame is a type of self-judgment that occurs when a client thinks, "I am bad" or "I am a bad person for having that thought." Feeling shame strikes at the client's sense of identity. "Beet greens are gross to some people. I can't like beet greens because they are gross. I am a bad person for liking beet greens." Shame can be such an issue in my day-to-day counseling sessions that I have found and created handouts to help explore the role of shame when it comes to food and eating.

COUNSELING ACTIVITY – WHAT IS SHAME?

DIRECTIONS: Read the definition of shame: "the intensely painful feeling or experience that we are flawed and, therefore, unworthy of connection or belonging."

Now call forth the Spirit of MI: Collaboration, how can I collaborate with my client who is experiencing shame?; Acceptance, how do I demonstrate acceptance when my client that is experiencing or expressing shame?; Compassion, how do I demonstrate compassion when my client is experiencing shame? And evocation, how do I call forth my client's own wisdom when she is experiencing shame? If you are struggling, come back to this Counseling Activity as the rest of this chapter may offer you more ideas and suggestions. Also consider journaling, creating a Thought Compass, or talking with your peers to explore and discover your answers to these questions.

GOING DEEPER
Debriefing Shame

After this activity regarding shame and MI, it is helpful to "debrief," or process, the experience.

1. Take a moment and write down what you liked about the shame/MI activity.

2. Now list what you would change in your counseling or self-talk. All awareness is helpful, even if you become aware of something unpleasant or unsettling about this shame/MI activity.

3. Stretch your skills by spending some time in reflection. Ask yourself the following four questions:

   - How have I observed this concept being presented?
   - How can I convey this concept using my own words and experiences?
   - Have I had an opportunity to teach this concept? If so, what resources do I currently have or use.
   - What steps am I taking to deepen and expand my counseling skills to reduce shame?

Paul Gilbert, PhD, describes shame as pathogenic and linked to two key processes. The first is the client's degree of self-directed hostility, contempt, and self-loathing. The second is the client's inability to generate feelings of self-directed warmth, soothing, and reassurance. As you can see, shame is big stuff.

The experience of shame — whether self-inflicted or a byproduct of a counseling session — creates the conditions for the client to seek other self-soothing coping tools, which may include food, eating, or self-harm behaviors. These are the exact behaviors that we as dietitians are trying to help the client with.

MOVING PAST SHAME: HOW MINDFULNESS CAN HELP

"Mindfulness is paying attention in a particular way: on purpose, in the present moment, nonjudgmentally.[16]" In a review of Mindfulness interventions, researchers Daphne Davis and Stephen Hayes[17] identified a number of benefits for both the client and the counselor. When a client engages in Mindfulness, there is improved regulation of emotions, decreased reactivity, and increased response flexibility, plus interpersonal and intrapersonal benefits. For the therapist, the benefits include empathy and compassion, and decreased stress and anxiety. Additional benefits are self-efficacy, patience, intentionality, gratitude, and body awareness.

Introducing Mindfulness is therapeutic and helpful to both the client and the dietitian. This fact is a beautiful gem to me, and it motivates me to practice Mindfulness — I get so much from the process! The trick is, Mindfulness is modeled, not taught. That means that nonjudgment needn't be a separate learning objective, or a box to check indicating "this task's done." Instead, it is a process infused into your counseling session.

CONNECTING

When I have presented this concept at such events as the Food and Nutrition Conference and Expo or the American Association of Diabetes Educators, many professionals have nodded in complete agreement — "Yes! Yes! Yes!" — and the excitement is radiating from their whole being. Then I look to the person right next to them: Furrowed brow, downturned mouth, and hunched back tell me that this person is frustrated, not sure she *should* change or *how to* change her counseling approach to include Mindfulness. Her frustration is palpable, and I connect so much to *that* dietitian because, as much as I love the concept, being mindful is effort. I've been in that seat, listening to someone talk about Mindfulness and thought, "I love this, but I don't get how to do it." The concept of Mindful Eating can feel remote to many professionals and to their clients. I want to bring it closer to you. The best way is to make Mindful Eating fresh again by helping you define the idea for yourself.

COUNSELING ACTIVITY – MAKE YOUR OWN PRINCIPLES OF MINDFUL EATING

DIRECTIONS: Create your personal definition, one that has meaning and resonance for you. This personal definition holds the wisdom and experience of your teachers, but with your own personal twist. Let your words and explanation reflect "what the wise would say." Use The Principles of Mindful Eating, created by The Center for Mindful Eating, to help you. It is available free on the website www.TheCenterForMindfulEating.org.

- Read The Principles of Mindful Eating or other definitions that reflect Mindful Eating.
- Circle the words that resonate within you, and cross off any words that bother you.
- Looking at the words that resonate, craft a paragraph that reflects the *Spirit* you want to convey in your counseling session. This activity can be helpful if you want to create a blog or business plan to promote Mindful Eating. Crafting a paragraph that reflects your thoughts and beliefs about Mindful Eating will help you distinguish yourself and your business from your restrictive-eating competition.
- Ask yourself if your paragraph promotes Collaboration, Acceptance, Compassion, and Evocation.

THE PRINCIPLES OF MINDFUL EATING

Mindful Eating is:

Allowing yourself to become aware of the positive and nurturing opportunities that are available through food selection and preparation by respecting your own inner wisdom.

Using all your senses in choosing to eat food that is both satisfying to you and nourishing to your body.

Acknowledging responses to food (likes, dislikes or neutral) without judgment.

Becoming aware of physical hunger and satiety cues to guide your decisions to begin and end eating.

GOING DEEPER
Debriefing the activity

1. Take a moment and write down what you liked about creating your own Principles of Mindful Eating activity.
2. Now list where else you can go to expand this personal Mindful Eating definition.
3. Spend some time in reflection, asking yourself the following four questions:

- How have I observed this concept being presented? Think about books, teachers, or research that supports these concepts.
- How can I convey this concept using my own words and experiences?
- How or when could I offer this concept to my clients?
- When I teach this, how will I use the feedback I have received to improve and expand my skills?

COUNSELING ACTIVITY – **THOUGHT COMPASS**

Mind Mapping is a technique that I have found helpful. I teach it in groups and as part of the Mindful Eating retreat that I lead. It is a tool developed by Tony Buzan, an English author and educational consultant. You can watch him teach it on YouTube in about an hour. He is very generous with his knowledge — an additional point of gratitude! What I like about Mind Mapping is that it gives people who are overwhelmed a way to organize their thoughts. It also helps people who are afraid to try new things a way to pause and see what is out there, to discover and consider new approaches. I also have found that, unlike journaling, Mind Mapping helps to organize your thoughts without creating a narrative, a huge advantage for clients who seem stuck. The intention of Mind Mapping is to simply see what "is." Mind Mapping promotes evocation — "calling forth" what the client already knows.

So how do you Mind Map? Below are the directions for a modified version of a Mind Mapping that I teach students and clients. I call this a Thought Compass because it is only offering an initial direction to become aware of. When using the Thought Compass, don't worry whether it is "right," just whether it is helpful or effective.

DIRECTIONS: In the center of a blank sheet of paper, draw a circle. From the circle, draw a line to the North, the South, the East and the West.

Now write a topic in the center of the circle. I wrote "Nonjudgment." *See Image 2*

Write a thought about Nonjudgement in the North, South, East, and West positions. *See Image 3*

As before, you can draw a line from each subtopic: Collaboration, Acceptance, Compassion and Evocation. Thought Compass until you have exhausted your ideas. *See Image 4*

I suggest that you create Thought Compass to help you explore all you know and have just learned. You might choose the following topics:

- Nonjudgment.
- Mindfulness.
- Shame.

For examples of completed Thought Compasses please visit www.megrette.com/coreconcepts.

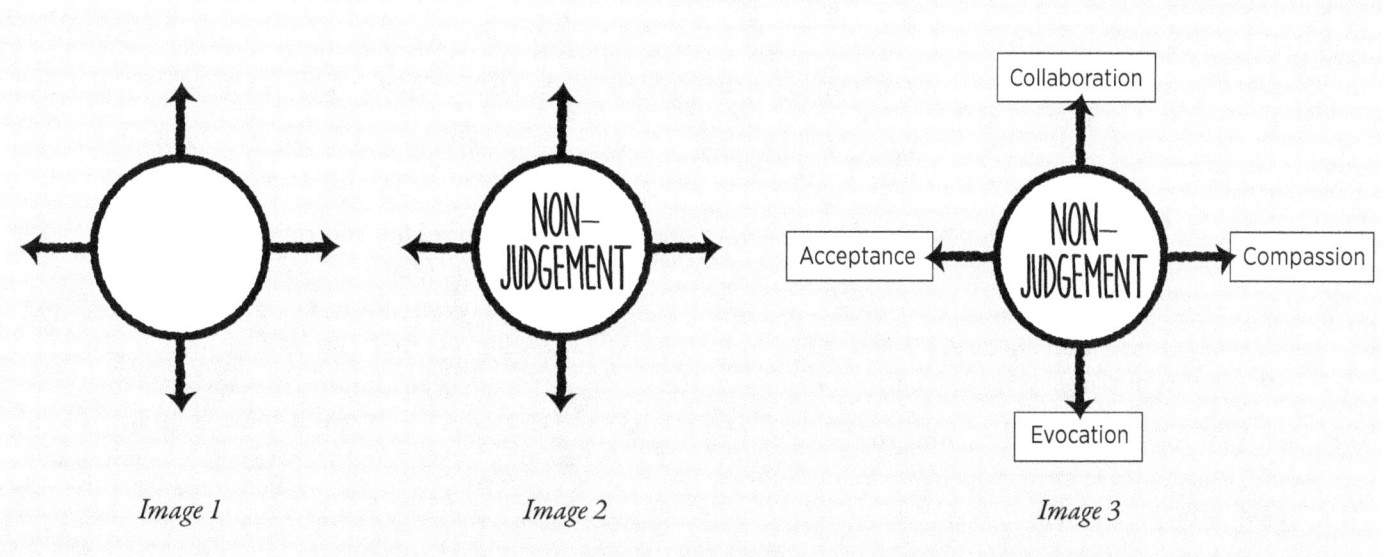

Image 1 *Image 2* *Image 3*

DIRECTIONS: Here is a partially completed Thought Compass. Take a few minutes and think of questions to ask yourself about what you know, what you have learned, where you can find more information about these four qualities

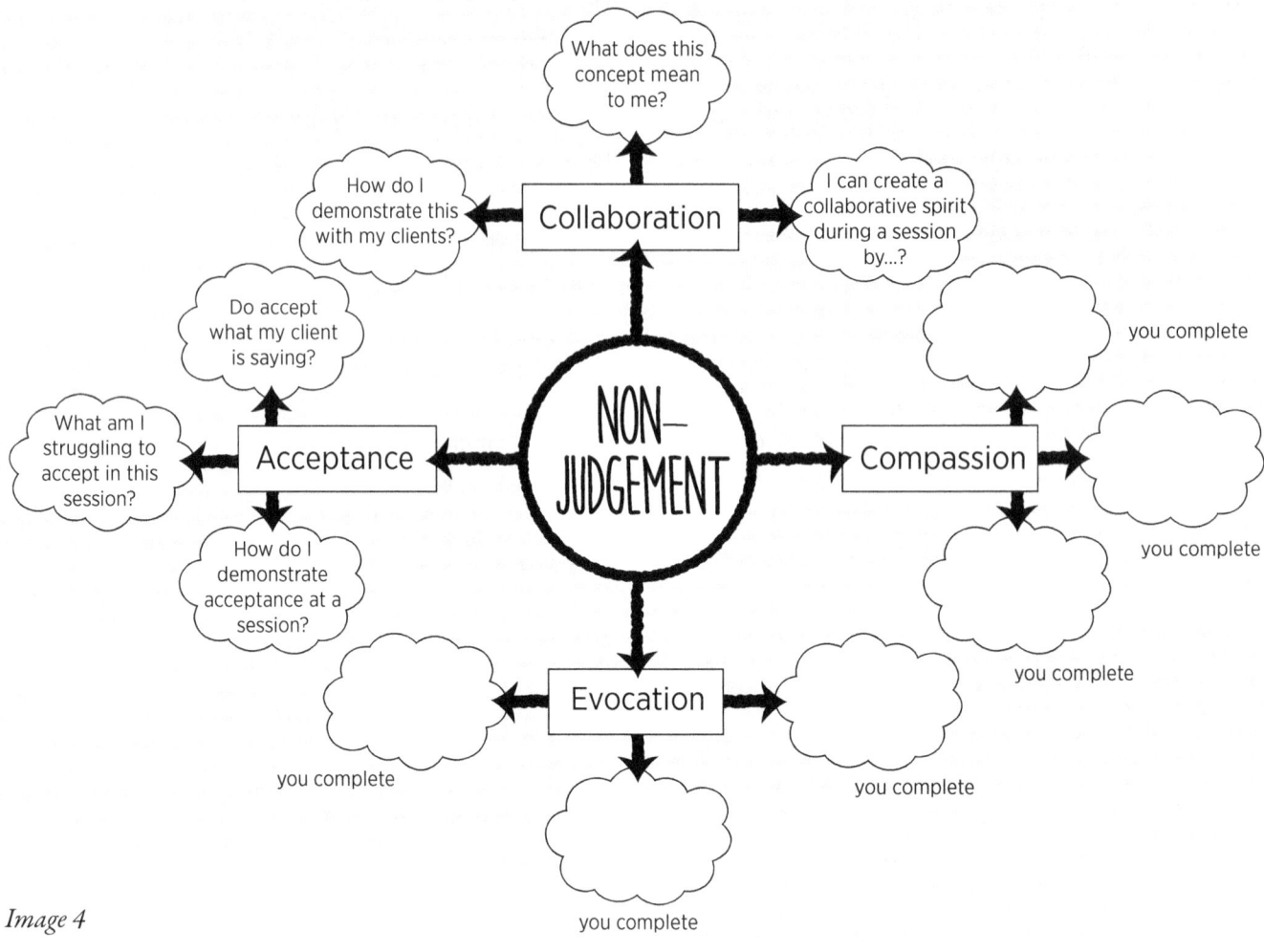

Image 4

GOING DEEPER
Debriefing a Thought Compass

Creating a Thought Compass is intended to be a fun and enjoyable experience. After you teach how to complete a Thought Compass, it is helpful to "debrief," or process, the experience with a class or another individual.

1. Take a moment and write down what your client liked about the Thought Compass activity.

2. Now list what the client didn't like about the activity. Remain nonjudgmental regarding the response. All awareness is helpful, even if you or your client become aware of something unpleasant about using a Thought Compass.

3. Using this feedback, think about what you want to change about the activity to make it more effective in your setting.

4. Stretch your skills by spending some time in reflection. Ask yourself the following four questions:

    - Have I observed this concept being presented?
    - Do I wish to I teach this concept? If I do, how can I use my own words and experiences?
    - When do I have an opportunity to teach this concept in a counseling or group session?
    - When I teach this, how will I use the feedback I have received to deepen and improve my counseling skills?

CONNECTING

Right before this book was about to be published a colleguage called me. She prefaced the call with the comment, "I wasn't sure I should tell you," which made my heart sink. I listened as she began to explain that she wasn't exactly sure "What Mindful Eating is?" As we talked I began to piece together the larger issue surrounding her concern. Mindful Eating isn't a thing or a check box that you do. Eating mindfully is a mental state that begins with the intention to let go of judgment. This nonjudgmental intention is a wish, if it is not supported with a practice to deepen your awareness, like meditation than it is unlikely the wish to be nonjudgmental will come true. So, in the mindful eating community, we talk about creating a formal awareness or reflection practice, to help you observe your judgment, nonjudgmentally! Yep, you are going to just notice when you were judgmental. Observing your judgmental thoughts and habits is hard, which is why you also cultivate a lot of self-compassion. These three steps are called the "Roots" of mindful eating and once you have practices these, mindful eating becomes much easier to experience, experiment with and espouse to others!

CHAPTER SUMMARY
The Spirit of Nonjudgment

HOORAY! Review the counseling tools you just learned.

- You have learned that nonjudgment can actually make you happier.

- You learned about the *Spirit* of MI, which is a great way to develop a nonjudgmental stance. The *Spirit* of MI promotes Collaboration, Acceptance, Compassion, and Evocation.

- You were introduced to the Thought Compass, an abbreviated form of Mind Mapping, which is a way to organize thoughts, understand, and resources.

OOPS! What are some struggles you might encounter?

- You unintentionally fall into a judgmental stance. I shared that being rushed and making faulty assumptions about my clients' motivations are my *typical* triggers.

- It is really hard to be with another person's suffering. This skill, to be with suffering in acceptance and collaboration, is challenging!

- You will actually never become free of judgment. Oh, my gosh! Wouldn't that be great to achieve? We mere humans simply need to focus on effort and progress, not the divine goal of perfection.

- Shame is a universal emotion that everyone has felt. It is defined as "the intensely painful feeling or experience that you are flawed and, therefore, unworthy of connection or belonging." You might recognize shame, but not be sure what to do about it.

TADA! Review the action steps of the chapter.

1. Consider whether it would be a helpful to have resource regarding shame when working with clients in an individual or a group setting.

2. Make Your Own *Principles of Mindful Eating* to help you connect and define your own beliefs about Mindful Eating.

3. Try A Thought Compass with the sample topics of nonjudgement, mindfulness and shame.

4. If curious, watch Tony Buzan explain the concept of Mind Mapping on YouTube.

EMPATHIZING - SITA

"I am sitting in a quiet space, and the thoughts in my head seem to just turn off, allowing me to hear, for the first time, the sounds all around. It is weird, you notice the sound of the room, the noises outside. With each inhaled breath, I am becoming more and more aware of what is present right now. I am loving meditating because I feel heard in a way that is both exciting and powerful. The thing is, my friends ask, "How was it?" This question leaves me without words, because I am unable to describe the experience. It happened, it changed me, yet I can't explain it to anyone. Am I normal?"

— Sita

CHAPTER 2
Meditation

"Only in the spaciousness of mind that is created by meditation can you see what your body, heart and mind are actually feeling and doing. This awareness shifts you out of automatic pilot. It gives you choice, and choice gives you freedom."

— Jan Chozen Bays, MD, "Mindful Eating"

Mindful Eating has its roots firmly planted in Mindfulness. To get the full benefit from Mindful Eating, a person has to practice engaging in nonjudgmental observation of the current situation – simply put, to meditate.

When professionals tell me that they want to learn about Mindful Eating, but that they don't have time to meditate, I know Mindful Eating isn't going to change their lives as it has mine. Do I believe that understanding the Core Concepts of Mindful Eating will be helpful? Absolutely! However, if your intention is to learn and not develop a mindfulness practice to support your journey, Mindful Eating will be a different experience for you than it is for a student with a deep and committed meditation practice. You may enjoy Mindful Eating, but you may never get to experience the sense of wonder and peace so many have discovered.

CONNECTING

When I first started to meditate, I was a bit annoyed with the whole experience. It seemed unnecessary, and painful, sitting still for 20 to 30 minutes, not to mention strangely removed from my stated goal, which was learning about Buddhism. However, I listened to my teachers, and I sat quietly, and "meditated" for many years. Upon reflection, I suspect I wasn't meditating, but simply sitting still thinking. It was time for reflection, and that by itself offers a lot of benefit. Then something happened. I was able to observe my direct experience nonjudgmentally! I was able to see my sensory experience as just that, an itch, or a noise. It wasn't actually very interesting, and it didn't need my attention. I was able to see my thoughts without getting carried away by them; I was able to watch my thoughts come and go, to see them as distinct from myself. I was able to witness my feelings, the fun and engaging feelings, as well as the darker feelings that are part of a rich life experience. I was able to be with all of these, and remain seated, remain still, nonreactive — and this experience changed me. As a result, my mind and, more important, my heart are bigger. This expansion of my thinking and my capacity to care feels profound and indescribable. It changed me by offering me insight into my own delusions, my own mental patterns, my own direct experience. And that remains a gift I cherish.

WHAT CAN MEDITATION DO FOR YOU?

More and more scientific benefits of meditation seem to be discovered weekly. The practice changes the brain as well as the cells in the body! Meditation is an effective coping mechanism for dealing with stresses of life. It can offer an intentional way to slow down. It is an effective way to cope with life's joys, celebrations, and endless possibilities. Meditation is a way to listen to all the information that resides within you. Meditation isn't for everyone. I know many professionals who practice yoga or have a committed practice of prayer and confession. These other contemplative practices are also effective and will likely offer the same benefit.

When a person in a session describes his contemplative practice or her attempts at meditation, then I know: This person is truly willing to change, to shake up his/her mind and grasp concepts seldom discussed in conversation, to see past the cravings and the desires for "thin" or "fast" or "easy" to the heart of the matter, to understand the suffering, unawareness, and self-harm. To these individuals, I would like to say, **Welcome!** The world needs your passion, vision, and help.

REFLECTING

As Chapter 1, "The Spirit of Nonjudgment," makes clear, Mindful Eating instructors are strongly encouraged to cultivate a regular practice of Mindfulness. While there are many ways to practice being present — through attentive listening, through awareness of our body and our environment while taking a walk, for example — I believe that meditation offers the most effective way to develop present-moment awareness. For that reason, this Mindful Eating book recommends that instructors learn and practice meditation. It will be especially important for you to have a meditation practice if you want to teach professionals. The Center for Mindful Eating offers *The Good Practice Guidelines*[18], which can help you understand this recommendation.

Meditation is important because your life involves emotions and situations that range from enjoyment and enrichment to suffering, poor health, shame, and struggle. Food and eating are not only about health and nutrition, but self-awareness and emotion as well. Meditation helps you explore these inner dimensions. The clarity and sense of ease that can be developed in meditation helps us to avoid judgment, which can overwhelm or oversimplify our relationship to food and eating. Over time, meditation helps us develop greater capacity for present-moment awareness and compassionate responses to life.

The following instruction is for you personally and offers help in encouraging participants of your Mindful Eating presentations to meditate as well. Several approaches are offered in this chapter.

WHAT IS MINDFULNESS?

What is mindfulness? What is meditation?

Mindfulness is not meditation. Meditation is not mindfulness. Mindfulness (as stated in the introduction) is the ability to become aware. Meditation is how you build or create awareness. It is important to clarify what I mean by these terms. Your understanding of mindfulness and meditation will evolve with practice and experience, for the purposes of this training, I will use commonly agreed-upon definitions.

Mindfulness refers to your ability to direct nonjudgmental awareness on purpose toward a particular aspect of experience or object of attention. Just as Motivational Interviewing promotes the Spirit of MI, meditation promotes the skills of a Mindful Eating professional. These skills include yet are not limited to:

- Nonjudgment and nonreactivity.
- Sustained attention or steady attention.
- A sense of direction or purpose or intent.
- A sense of what is "skillful" or helpful and ethical.

Mindfulness can have a broad or narrow scope or "object." Traditionally, you develop Mindfulness in these realms:

- Of self (body, mind, action).
- Of others.
- Of your environments.
- Of life or reality.

These qualities contrast with ordinary waking awareness, in which you are often jumping from topic to topic and filled with reactions and judgments to most everything you come in contact with.

Meditation helps you cultivate mindfulness and to know your mind more thoroughly. It is the "lab work" for becoming connected and aware. Like Mindful Eating, not all meditations will be enjoyable. Don't worry if sometimes meditating is more challenging.

In the next chapter, you will see that your struggle is my struggle and that we are connected by this common experience. If you are struggling to start a meditation practice, I would like to encourage you to get additional support. The Center for Mindful Eating offers community meditations, and there are many additional resources listed at the end of this book.

The types of meditation most supportive to Mindful Eating come under the umbrella of "mindfulness." Recalling the definition from Jon Kabat-Zinn, "Mindfulness means paying attention in a particular way, on purpose, in the present moment, and nonjudgmentally." These forms of meditation calm and focus your minds, as well as increase self-awareness. They help you to concentrate and to direct our mind, making the mind more pliable and more aware of choices. People from around the world have developed meditations that support their faiths and cultures. I would like to acknowledge these and also clearly state that it is not the intention of this book to become a definitive meditation resource, which is why this book is focusing on mindfulness meditations.

A number of meta-analysis and comparative review articles have been published which conclude moderate evidence supporting mindfulness meditation to improve anxiety, depression, and pain.[19] Programs which included a meditation component, such as MBSR had the strongest effect on psychological well-being.[20] Meditation can also benefit a person personally and spiritually, yet the boundary between these two may be interwoven. Looking specifically at using kindness based meditations shows moderate strength of evidence in decreasing self-reported depression, increasing mindfulness, compassion, and self-compassion. Meditation was more effective at generating positive emotions when compared to relaxation.[21]

Ways of using your mind in meditation include:

- Noticing, observing, taking note, sensing, listening, being present to, focusing on, attending, etc. (It may be helpful in your teaching of Mindful Eating to use these guiding words, not only for guided meditation, but also for training the mind in nonjudgment.)

What are the benefits of mindfulness meditation practice?

- Since a person will always want to be aware, there is a shift in the words used to describe meditation. It isn't an activity you complete, but it is one that you practice. This idea of creating a meditation practice is to acknowledge that practicing becoming mindful will help you to have greater choice in all arenas of your life. Therefore, your practicing mindful awareness becomes your "Practice."

- Practice helps you to respond to inner and outer stimuli with considered intent, rather than with automatic reactivity. People who practice meditation are often better able to enjoy the pleasures and meet the challenges of life.

- Practice helps you improve your physical and mental health. Physical effects include improved sleep, reduced stress, lower blood pressure. Mental and emotional effects include relief for anxiety, depression, obsession-compulsion, and eating disorders, and increased capacity for self-regulation.[22]

STARTING A MEDITATION

How do you begin to meditate? Meditation can begin in any position. Traditionally, a person sits on the floor on a hard cushion called a zafu, which provides more space for your legs to be folded comfortably beneath you. The intent is to have your spine straight.

- Posture — straight spine, regardless of whether you sit on the floor or in a chair, a.k.a. a dignified posture.

- Body awareness — sit comfortably and keep your mind focused on your body.

- Locate the breath, resting your awareness on the breath.

- Try to meditate for 20 minutes. You may need to work up to this duration.

- Short option: 3-minute breath awareness.

- If you or your client suffers from high anxiety, it might be better starting with present awareness outside the body. This would mean focusing on the sounds and sensations that are happening in the room or the world outside before attempting to listen to the body.

- If you or your client is ready, bring in some awareness of body and body sensations by focusing on the breath. With additional training, individuals may choose to observe thoughts and feelings.

LEADING A MEDITATION

- When including a meditation as part of a nutrition program, keep the session short, 3-10 minutes.

- When teaching or leading a meditation, aim to lead a full 20-to-30-minute sit.

- If desired, you can choose a guided meditation, using imagery to refocus the mind, such as, "The body is like a mountain or earth," or "Feelings, like water in a stream, flow on by," or "The mind is like the clear blue sky where there is nothing to grasp or hold onto." A sample script has been provided.

- Have bells, chimes, or an auditory way to signal that the session has ended.

FOUR TYPES OF MINDFULNESS MEDITATIONS

A3D Breathing Space

Sit comfortably (or you can stand or lie down). You may close the eyes or keep them open, but with eyes unfocused and gazing slightly downward.

A for Awareness or Attention

- Be conscious of your attention and awareness.
- Bring attention to what you notice now. Notice that it changes second by second.
- Continue just noticing ... just noticing ... whatever comes into awareness.

3 for 3-dimensional: body, heart, mind

- Bring attention and awareness to your body.
- To your heart (or emotion or mood).
- To your mind or thoughts.
- Notice what is going on — no need to change or adjust or interpret in any way.
- Simply notice.

D for Drop in or Deepen

- Continue being aware of body, heart, and mind.
- Continue being conscious of attention.
- Drop into a deeper sense of your experience, simply being aware of what is "underneath" all the changing details.

Practice A3D breathing space for 3 minutes or more any time you wish. (But not while driving or operating machinery!)

Mindful Awareness in Three Stages

Sit comfortably with back upright, so that you feel stable
and have good contact with your chair or supports.

1. Settle into body awareness. Scan through the body gently and gradually to "arrive" more fully in your posture. Notice what is present, allowing for any spontaneous adjustments or letting go that occurs as you give attention to different parts of the body.

2. Locate the breath. Focus on the movement of the body with the breath. Tune in to that part of the body where you feel the breath coming and going.

3. Sit and breathe. Notice the subtleties and details of the body sitting and the body breathing – the rise and fall, the flow of air, the in and out – and allow all competing thoughts, emotions, and distractions to move to the background, "anchoring" your awareness to the specific sensations of the body sitting, the body breathing.

Practice Mindful Awareness of the Body and Breath for as
long as you wish – 20-50 minutes is recommended.

Kindness and Compassion Meditation

- Arrive in your seat, become aware of the body, and anchor with the breath.
    - Notice the body and breath as a whole.
    - Notice mood, feel tone.
    - Notice thoughts.

- Be aware of the coming and going of thoughts, feelings, sensations as complete experience, not grasping, just experiencing, as though listening attentively to a stream that flows by endlessly.

- Cultivate a kind, nonjudging, (forgiving) attitude toward whatever presents itself.

- Surround whatever arises with kindness. This means "being with" the total experience in a radical way. It means avoiding any temptation to "process" or "interpret" or "manage" what you are aware of. It means gently setting aside any temptation to judge or criticize or deny what arises.

- Allow images or brief scenarios to arise without following them in detail. Simply acknowledge and "be with" the situations and experiences of your life and your being. This deep acknowledgment is the seed of compassion.

- Bring another person to mind, if you wish, and sit with them in your heart as though deeply listening to their experience of life in all its richness of joy and sorrow, ease and pain, success and failure. Kindness and compassion can hold it all. Just "be with" and relax any urge to "do" anything.

- Finally, relax all specific imaginings and just sit with a sense of the body, of the breath, and especially of your heart area.

Traditional Metta Bhavna Meditation

In traditional Buddhist metta, or loving-kindness meditation, one brings to mind people who represent different kinds of relationships to us. In succession:

1. A teacher, mentor, or benefactor.
2. Oneself.
3. A good friend.
4. Someone we hardly know and feel neutral toward.
5. Someone we have difficulty with.
6. We then bring all together and have a sense of kindness, respect, and care toward all equally, expanding to include all beings whatsoever.

Traditional "wishes" of loving-kindness are:

May (he, she, I, you, all beings) be safe and free from harm.

May (he, she, I, you, all beings) be well and at ease.

May (he, she, I, you, all beings) be happy.

May (he, she, I, you, all beings) be fulfilled (awakened, become Enlightened).

This is a variation of the Metta Bhavna that resonates within me, but you can make your own wishes.

May (he, she, I, you, all beings) be well.

May (he, she, I, you, all beings) have access to the conditions to ease suffering.

May (he, she, I, you, all beings) be free of pain.

May (he, she, I, you, all beings) be happy.

Meditations Script

MINDFUL EATING MEDITATION
By Marge Morris M.Ed., RD

Welcome. We will be meditating for [x] minutes. Find your seat and settle into a comfortable position. Take 3 deep breaths, then return to normal breathing, allowing your feet to rest comfortably on the floor with your spine erect but not tense. Be here now, observing your breath, allowing the in and out breath to flow naturally.

At the end of the next exhale, notice the space after the exhale and just before the next inhale. As breathing continues, feel into the quiet energy of this space.

If your mind wanders, gently return your focus to the breath and that quiet space between the exhale and inhale. As the breathing continues, relax and become more in-tune to this quiet energy. Breathing in ... breathing out.

[Gently offer centering words through the meditation every 5 minutes or so]

As we near the end of our session, expand your awareness to include sound. In a few moments, you will hear 3 chimes, and this will conclude our session. Then gently open your eyes and move into the rest of your day.

Meditations Script

10-MINUTE MEDITATION
By Barbara Boothby, MS, RD

Welcome. We will be meditating for [x] minutes. We will start an awareness of breathing meditation.

Take a moment to get comfortable.

Now, see if there is anything else you need to feel supported.

Allow yourself to feel grounded … to the chair, the cushion.

On your next inhale, invite the breath into the spaces between your vertebrae, cushioning them, elongating your spine, supporting you.

On your next exhale, allow your shoulders to roll back and down a little bit, as if they are gently heading toward your back pockets.

Now, imagine the crown of your head being held up gently by a thread.

Notice what it feels like to sit like this.

Now, take in a deep breath, a breath of gratitude for being here, in this moment.

Deepen your next exhale a bit. You might even say "Ah" if you wish as you exhale, and as you do so, release anything you don't want to be holding onto right now. Repeat this 1 or 2 more times if you would like. Then, allow the breath to return to its natural rhythm.

Breathing in. Breathing out.

You can use this cycle of the breath as an anchor for your awareness. As you focus your awareness on the breath, allow any thoughts or sensations to recede into the background.

Not trying to change anything.

Not trying to stop anything from happening.

Not trying to make anything happen.

We are allowing a space where we can be with whatever arises in each moment — be it thought, or emotion, or body sensation — allowing, with the intention not to engage anything.

Breathing in. Breathing out.

[To end the meditation]

As this meditation draws to a close, expand your awareness to take in the sensations in your body, the sounds of the room. In a moment, you will hear the sound of a bell. When you can no longer hear the bell, open your eyes slowly when you are ready. Gently move your body in a way that feels good to you.

(Ring bell)

COUNSELING ACTIVITY

Consider recording your own voice as you read the meditation scripts. Use this self-recording as a way to start your class, group, or personal practice. You can also have clients read and record their own meditation script to support an emerging meditation practice.

GOING DEEPER
Debriefing a meditation

Creating a meditation practice is different from teaching meditation. This book does not provide adequate instruction for you to teach meditation to clients. Additional instruction, training, and practice are required. However, if you are experienced in meditation and you wish to include some aspect of meditation in your session, class, or group, you will need to provide specific instruction. It is my belief that after you teach meditation, it is helpful to "debrief," or process, the experience with a class or individual.

1. Take a moment and write down what you or your client noticed about the meditation.

2. Now list what you or your client would change or found challenging about the meditation. Remain nonjudgmental regarding the response. All awareness is helpful, even if there is awareness of something unpleasant about meditation.

3. Try to summarize the Pros and Cons of meditation. Allow this summary to inform your teaching.

4. Stretch your skills by spending some time in reflection. Ask yourself the following four questions:
   - How have I observed meditation being presented?
   - How can I convey the value, purpose, and benefits of mediation using my own words and experiences?
   - When would I have an opportunity to teach this concept?
   - Where do I get feedback to improve my skill at teaching meditation? What options are available for me to learn and expand my meditation skills?

COUNSELING A DEBRIEFING SESSION WITH CLIENTS OR IN A GROUP

Meditation can be a powerful tool. Many people enjoy meditation because it offers them some much-needed space to relax and distress. However, meditation is not always welcome, pleasant, or easy. As a teacher, give space for your client's meditation experience to be anything, from delight to dread. There is no right or wrong outcome to mediation. The outcome is simply present.

After a meditation instruction and activity has been completed, debrief and relate the experience back for the learner. This is when the real learning takes place. Allow adequate time to complete this step.

USING A MI TECHNIQUE TO DEBRIEF YOUR COUNSELING ACTIVITIES

Motivational Interviewing offers some wonderful tools to help your counseling. One foundational tool, and one of my favorites, is the mnemonic OARS, which stands for:

O: Ask ***open-ended questions***. Let your questions be gentle and curious in order to learn the details of how the clients sees a behavior as part of his life.

A: ***Affirm*** the answers that you hear. Reflections are nonjudgmental and avoid criticizing or blaming. You, as a counselor do not have to believe the reflection for these to be accurate, empathic and effective. For example: "You are seeing the benefit of meditation, even if you can't place it into words."

R: ***Reflect*** back the connections and emotions that individuals offer. Recognizing specific strengths and linking them to support your client's behaviors can help move her towards change. For example: "You still want to meditate."

S: ***Summarize*** the learning that was discovered by meditation. Show that you are listening carefully, which can help you emphasize and guide your client towards her goals.

Let's explore how this might look in a group or counseling session:

- Start by expressing gratitude. This is typically done by saying, "Thank you for … [meditating with me, your time, your attention, your willingness to try something different]…"
- Next, focus on what was good about the experience. A possible script:
  - "What did you ***enjoy*** about this meditation?" After you have heard from the individuals in the room, acknowledge their responses.
  - Next ask, "What was hard or that you disliked about the activity?" Maintain an open, curious stance in your review of the benefits and challenges of meditation. Give equal importance to what was challenging as what was beneficial during the sit.
  - This small but important step of identifying ambivalence will be helpful later in your counseling when you move to facilitating change. You may wish to keep a list of benefits/challenges to meditation for your group to review.
- Thank everyone for sharing, and proceed to the benefits of meditation that you would like to share.
- You can also see if there are any unspoken needs or questions about meditation.
  - Summarize the experience. *"Thank you for participating. Most of you enjoyed the experience. There were some unanswered questions, like what is the best position to sit in, and some challenges, such as when should you meditate. I am confident we can address these going forward."*
- You can ask if people are interested in meditating on their own. If they are, determine what supports are needed to assist. This might be phone apps like Insight Timer, or meditation scripts or recordings.

RETURNING TO THE FIRST SECTION OF THIS CHAPTER: EMPATHIZING

... The thing is, my friends ask, "How was it?" This question leaves me without words, because I am unable to describe the experience. It happened, it changed me, yet I can't explain it to anyone. Am I normal?

— Sita

A common occurrence for both the professional and the individual in Mindful Eating is having a profound experience that they cannot express in words. If this has happened to you, chances are it can happen to your clients.

When this happens, coach yourself by acknowledging that you have had an experience that it is hard for you to describe ... **at this moment**. There is nothing wrong, there is nothing to worry about, you are processing the experience of listening to yourself and possibly feeling heard.

It is common to wonder:

- Is this NORMAL?
- Is this a GOOD sign?
- Did I do something wrong?
- Should I be worried?

Review your coaching skills, and listen to yourself. It may be helpful to identify whether the experience was Pleasant, Neutral, or Unpleasant. Remain nonjudgmental, and ask open-ended questions to promote understanding about the experience. Affirm the experience: "Many people find that after a meditation, they cannot fully articulate the experience." By asking an open-ended question, such as, "What concerns you about this particular experience?" you can discover whether there is a specific worry.

Remain in the present moment with the meditation experience. Resist reading into the experience or creating expectations about future meditations. Simply affirm that this meditation was hard to describe, that it has [increased/decreased] your interest in having another meditation.

When I am faced with this situation, I often need to take a deep breath and add a dose of self-compassion before I focus on my ability to sit with my own uncertainty. It is lovely to pretend that I know what is best, and what to do for my clients at every moment. Mindfulness and Mindful Eating counseling challenges this wish. If you are struggling to welcome uncertainty in your life, or in your counseling practice, you are not alone! This is the hard stuff because you are acknowledging that there are no guarantees, that the outcome is uncertain.

When you pair empathy with pure nonjudgmental acceptance at the heart of all mindfulness and Mindful Eating programs, something magical seems to happen — you are a witness not only to yourself, but also to your participants. The experience of being a "witness" has felt very sacred to me. I remind myself that I was invited to hear, watch, observe, offer support, and rejoice in a life that is unfolding.

COUNSELING ACTIVITY – **THOUGHT COMPASS**

Consider completing a Thought Compass to help you understand your meditation experience. Begin with the blank Thought Compass. Consider what you know about meditation. Pull out four key aspects of the meditation to explore and write in the North, South, East, and West points of the Thought Compass. Examples include finding a different sitting position, struggling to make time to meditate, wanting to have a timer, or observations you remember. The sky's the limit, and it is 100% OK to create a Thought Compass that you don't fully understand or that doesn't make any sense ... yet!

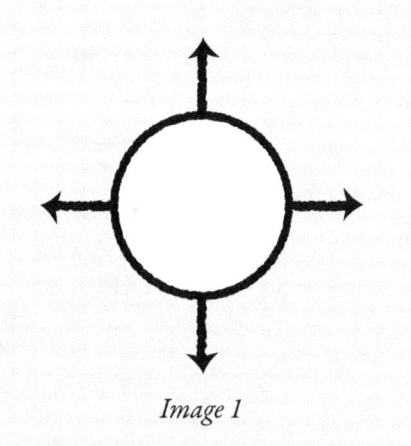

Image 1

CHAPTER SUMMARY
Meditation

HOORAY! Here are counseling tools and resources to help you.

- There are many meditations to try. Start with yourself.
- Record these meditations and listen to them, or play the audio for a group or client.
- There are other wonderful free meditations to explore, including the resources at:
  - The Center for Mindful Eating website.
  - Insight Timer, a smartphone application.
  - See Additional Resources at the end of the book for more ideas.

OOPS! What are the struggles you might encounter?

- As professionals, it is easy to forget that we are in touch with an area of life that includes enjoyment and enrichment, but also suffering, poor health, shame, and struggle.
- You may not be able to articulate the experience that arises when you meditate. This is normal. Being with our experience, including our uncertainty, is an important skill.
- Mindfulness is not meditation. Meditation is not mindfulness. Mindfulness (as stated in the introduction) is the ability to become aware. Meditation is how you build or create awareness.
- There are many different types of meditations for various reasons. Some will resonate with you more than others will.
- There isn't a "good" or "bad" meditation. Continue to practice, holding a nonjudgmental stance while learning to meditate.
- Being "good" at meditation isn't the desired outcome of a practice. The intent of meditation is to develop a regular and consistent practice. Your ability to meditate will be what it is. Resist the urge to judge/label it.

TADA! Here are the activities and action steps of the chapter.

- Meditations for you to try:
  - A3D Breathing Space.
  - Mindful Awareness in Three Stages.
  - Kindness and Compassion Meditation.
  - Traditional Metta Bhavna Meditation.
  - 2 Meditation Scripts:
- Identify ways to debrief your experience with meditation. These include journaling, using the Thought Compass, creating lists of helpful and unhelpful aspects of meditation as a way to stay motivated to practice.
- Complete a Thought Compass of your experience with meditation as a way to evoke or call forth what you know about mediation.
- Seek additional training in meditation before offering this to your clients!

EMPATHIZING - LINDA

"Yes, I am trying to engage in self-kindness in a more consistent way. I am choosing to do this in a number of ways, none of which I am sure will work. In all honesty, I am not 100% sure what self-kindness is or isn't. I see people talking about it like a diet, you know, drink this in the morning and 'poof' you are kind, or something. I get frustrated because it feels like the high road, noble and good, but for me, it is simply frustrating because I don't know what self-kindness is!"

— Linda

Chapter 3
Defining Self-Kindness

"You are the person who knows yourself most intimately. Therefore you are the person who can take care of yourself in the best ways. Become your best friend, and care for yourself as you would your best friend."
— Jan Chozen Bays, MD, "Mindful Eating"

Self-kindness, what Buddhism calls "metta," is part of a larger concept of self-compassion. A typical challenge that you, the professional, will face is when individuals confuse the concept of self-kindness with specific actions or diets. In this chapter, we will explore how Mindful Eating can help clients set the intention for self-kindness and self-care, allowing him/her to establish a sustainable model of change, instead of a punishing, guilt-creating cycle of restrictive eating. At the end of this chapter, you will find the tools and techniques that are used in meditation, self-compassion theory, and motivational interviewing for promoting the concept of self-kindness.

Pause for a moment and consider self-kindness. How would you describe it? The concept of self-kindness can be understood, but verbalizing it to another person proves challenging. Even harder than defining self-kindness is identifying it. Self-kindness is an internal consideration that is individualized and related to a specific situation. This means you can't say that a specific behavior is or isn't kind, because you don't know the individual's thoughts or the context that led to the behavior. For example, eating when you are not hungry may or may not be kind. If food would not be available later, it may be a kind act. If the decision to eat was a way of avoiding working or completing a project, it still may or may not be kind for lots of reasons. The point is YOU, the counselor cannot determine whether an action is or isn't kind. If you are agreeing with this logic, you are likely thinking, Dang-it! This awareness and assessment that an action is or isn't kind has to be made by the client. If this rings true to you, you are likely thinking, Double dang-it! How do I do that? Deep breath. Looking at change in this way is hard, but you are not alone. You already know about the importance of nonjudgmental stance discussed in Chapter 1. You already know that meditation can help open the mind and identify behavioral patterns. Now the next thing to learn is the role of self-kindness.

This inability to place self-kindness into a box creates a lot of confusion and doubt about what self-kindness actually is. For most of us, self-kindness defies definition! Vietnamese Buddhist monk Thich Nhat Hanh says, "There is no way to peace, peace is the way." You can use this same reasoning to understand the path to self-kindness. "There is no way to self-kindness, self-kindness is the way."

If there is no way to self-kindness except by engaging in self-kindness, you may be wondering how to articulate this — not only to yourself, but also in a session. It appears that the action, self-kindness, is also the benefit, self-kindness, which becomes a circular definition. Adding to the struggle is that self-kindness lacks the marketing appeal of weight loss or of getting into shape, because self-care is unique to each person — making it impossible to define! Oh, triple dang-it!

REFLECTING

Self-kindness is a root of Mindfulness and Mindful Eating, and it is part of a larger concept called self-compassion. Focusing solely on self-kindness in a session can make Mindful Eating feel elusive, remote, incomprehensible to many participants. As we heard from Linda, self-kindness may seem like "... the high road, all noble and good," but it can also feel pretty frustrating when a client has never taken time to explore what self-kindness is to them!

Many clients think that self-kindness is an action, like exercise or weight loss. It may feel easier for a client to focus on eating less sugar, avoiding junk food, losing weight, or eating a specific diet than to wrap her head around something "all noble and good." Keep in mind that these goals are HOW a client wants to express self-kindness. Many dietitians who want to teach Mindful Eating struggle when their clients express a desire that might sound like restrictive eating, such as "I have cut out sugar" or "I am focusing on the calories of foods." They wonder: "Should I tell the client what to do?"

Pause, and let yourself not react to these statements. Instead, try to understand what is driving the desire to "cut out sugar" or "focus on calories." This pause may help you see that the action is *how* the client wants to express self-care. It isn't the whole story, but only a part of a much larger story. To guide the client toward the present moment is asking the client to explore what her experience is to "cut out sugar" or "focus on calories." Mindful Eating is focusing on the clients' experience and often doesn't need comment or judgment.

Unfortunately, your client may be craving the *reassurance* that they are moving in a direction of self care and this can create a counseling struggle. Again, pause and try to help the client see the larger question, which is do these thought and behaviors support the larger goal of self-kindness. This could be done by asking the client to "walk me through how you would make a food decision with the intention to eat less sugar." Mindful Eating is effective when you listen to the client's underlying intention while staying firmly in the present moment. I continue to find that using Motivational Interviewing tools and techniques is the most effective counseling method for proceeding nonjudgmentally.

SELF-KINDNESS IS NOT A THING

Mindfulness and Mindful Eating are rooted in many Buddhist teachings, which describe this quality of self-kindness as "loving-kindness," or metta — defined as benevolence, loving-kindness, friendliness, amity, friendship, good will, kindness, and active interest in others. When these qualities are directed toward oneself, a person will begin to experience self-kindness. Some individuals confuse self-kindness with self-indulgence, which is having these qualities for ourselves, but not extending them toward others. When these qualities are expressed to oneself as well as others, in equal measure, self-indulgence becomes kindness.

CONNECTING

For years, no matter what I read or who I talked to, every time someone said "self-kindness," I would hear "selfish" or "self-indulgent." It was this little quirk in my head that motivated me to learn to deepen my meditation practice. The instructor was wonderful. But again, every time the word "self-kindness" was spoken, I heard "selfish." I bet my reaction was so obvious that my face might have contracted, into something of a prune, with pursed lips, as if I had tasted something sour. My childhood upbringing told me that "selfish" was the ultimate insult you might use to describe someone! There I was, in the kitchen of the Buddhist center, a lovely man chatting with me, when the conversation turned to self-kindness. He was very experienced in meditation and just happened to be a psychologist. Seeing my pursed lips and pained expression at the mere mention of "self-kindness" was his first clue that something was a bit off for me. When I expressed my idea that engaging in self-kindness was selfish, I think it removed all doubt. He listened, then offered me the following activity, which helped me understand this concept very quickly. I loved the activity, and since then, I have done it hundreds of times in my office with clients.

COUNSELING ACTIVITY – **SELF-KINDNESS = EQUAL**

To begin, make your hands into two fists and hold them in front of you, about chest high. Your fists represent you and another person. They are equal. This is how you can imagine self-kindness. You will do for yourself as you would for another person. Self-kindness means equal or the same.

Now raise the fist representing yourself, so it is above the other person. This is selfishness. Selfishness and self-indulgence are when you regard yourself above another person.

Now move the fist representing yourself below the other person. This is when you let other people take advantage of your good nature, and you find yourself feeling more empty and depleted than refreshed.

Now, place your fists so they are level again, and remind yourself, "I am are not selfish when I care for myself. I am expressing self-kindness." When you let your kindness be expressed to all things equally, it becomes a way to see and evaluate self-compassion: "Would I do this for others and not myself?"

GOING DEEPER
Debriefing Self-Kindness Activity

When you set the counseling conditions to explore the concept of self-kindness, remember to pause and evaluate what was helpful and where more exploration was needed. This can be done by:

1. Taking a moment to write down what you or your client liked about the activity.

2. List what you or your client would change. Remain nonjudgmental regarding the response. All awareness is helpful, even if you or your client become aware of something unpleasant or unsettling about the concept of self-kindness.

3. Stretch your skills by spending some time in reflection. Ask yourself the following four questions:

    - How have I observed the concept of self-kindness and self-compassion presented?
    - How can I convey this concept using my own words and experiences?
    - Have I had an opportunity to present self-kindness in a session, class, or group? Or to model this concept?
    - How will I use the feedback I have received from teaching this concept to improve or deepen my ability to communicate self-kindness?

COUNSELING ACTIVITY: DEFINING SELF-KINDNESS

DIRECTIONS: Write down what the concept of self-kindness means to you.

Now, with this definition, take a few minutes, and list three examples of how you express self-kindness. If you would like to add some difficulty, don't attach your expression of self-kindness to appearance. For example: Getting my hair cut is appearance-based.

Example 1: This example requires very little effort

Example 2: This example requires a moderate amount of effort

Example 3: This example requires much more difficult and takes the most amount of effort

At the end of this chapter, please revisit this activity to see if your answers would change or might be modified in some way after exploring the concept of self-kindness. The more you explore self-kindness, the clearer and easier acts of self-kindness become.

SELF-KINDNESS IS A MENTAL CONCEPT AND AN EMOTIONAL EXPERIENCE

As a mental concept, self-kindness is part of the thinking process. This means you can talk about being "kind." You can label kindness: "Oh, that is kind." You can judge or evaluate kindness: "Oh, that is the kindest thing I have ever seen!" or "He is so much kinder than most people." These are all examples of your thinking about kindness.

You can also feel kindness. When an action is kind, it hits you, you might feel emotions filling up your chest. Maybe you might tear up, becoming *verklempt*. This experience of feeling a kindness is much different than thinking about kindness. Mick — a physician with type 1 diabetes whom I assist with supporting our growing adult type 1 diabetes community — talks often about the "13-inch journey." This is what he calls the path from our heads to our hearts. The 13-inch journey is when an idea or concept goes from our head (thinking about self-kindness) to our hearts (experiencing self-kindness).

HOW TO MAKE THE 13-INCH JOURNEY

Wouldn't it be nice if there was a single way to connect our heads and our hearts with kindness? If a single path isn't possible, maybe we could have a few options — instead of the thousands of choices that are available both large and small every day. I am not sure if it is a blessing or a curse, but there is not one way, one step, or one action that makes a person kind or creates self-kindness. The path to self-kindness is self-created.

Why? Self-kindness is part of something much greater — self-compassion. Researcher Kristin Neff[23] explains that there are three parts to self-compassion: self-kindness, common humanity, and mindfulness (*Table 1*). We have already explored the concept of self-kindness. Let's move our understanding to our common humanity.

Table 1.

3 aspects of self-compassion, 3 situations calling for self-compassion	
Self-kindness	Self-critical
Common Humanity	Isolation
Mindfulness	Overidentification

COMMON HUMANITY

Neff identifies the second fundamental element of self-compassion as the recognition of the common human experience. This awareness of interconnection – that we are all in this together and that all of our lives are intertwined — helps to distinguish self-compassion from mere self-acceptance or self-love. "Compassion," Neff explains, "literally means 'to suffer with,' which implies a basic mutuality in the experience of suffering." The human experience is something we all share; it is imperfect and painful and inescapable.

MINDFULNESS

The concept of Mindfulness has been touched on and will be covered in more depth further on in this book. For the purpose of this chapter, Neff says that the value of mindfulness is "...the clear seeing and nonjudgmental acceptance of what's occurring in the present moment — facing up to reality, in other words. The idea is that we need to see things as they are, no more, no less, to respond to our current situation in the most compassionate — and therefore effective — manner."

To me, reading those words feels like a big hug. It resonates with a level of truth that I find very comforting. Mindfulness therefore is a path to self-kindness and self-compassion.

SITUATIONS THAT CALL FOR SELF-COMPASSION

SELF-CRITICAL

The opposite of having self-compassion is being self-critical. The self-critical voice is often so prevalent that a person is almost deaf to the rapid, snarking, biting comments that play in his head. These self-critical messages erode the foundation of self-compassion. To counter the self-critical voice requires the repeated application of self-kindness and self-compassion.

ISOLATION

It is easy, even tempting, to focus on our shortcomings without taking the larger human picture into account. When this happens, our perspective gets very small and narrow. We become absorbed in our own feelings of insufficiency and insecurity. This small space we have created confines us to a prison of self-loathing – and we are all alone there. Isolation calls for self-kindness and self-compassion.

OVERIDENTIFICATION

Have you noticed, sometimes, when you think about some typical comments that they just don't make sense? For example, have you ever said, "I'm sorry that it's raining out." The comment could be interpreted as you somehow feeling responsible for the rain. (Hopefully, most people assume that you are expressing empathy that I have been caught in the rain!) We mindlessly say things that assume responsibility for circumstances beyond our control. Slowly, we feel personally responsible for them. Wanting to change a situation that is beyond your control is lovely, but at some point, it shifts to overidentification. The feeling that "I caused this problem" becomes self-blame, which leads to other emotions that disconnect a person from self-compassion. Overidentification calls for self-kindness and self-compassion.

REFLECTING SELF-KINDNESS FOR YOUR CLIENTS

As you experience a client's desire to engage in self-kindness and self-care, you can acknowledge this desire by reflecting back to him what is present. Reflections are an important counseling tool, and there are two types that are especially helpful: Simple and Complex.

- A simple reflection of Linda's comment: "You don't want to feel uncomfortable in your body" or "You want to understand what kindness is."

- A complex reflection of Linda's comment: "You are afraid that your inability to lose weight is harming your health" or "Not understanding what kindness is makes you feel uneducated, and you are too embarrassed to tell anyone you are not sure what kindness is all about."

Offering simple reflections helps the client know that you are listening. Offering complex reflections helps the client know you understand the larger issue, which is often linked to self-kindness and self-care.

Our society offers a lot of advice on how to take care of yourself. This advice is often conveyed in a black or white message that squeezes a confusing and complex issue into a headline or a Tweet. These reductive messages nourish the fear of failure, making it difficult to start the change process. Reflection helps clients hear their own fears and their own reasons not to change. Reflection can also help to identify the desire to change and to acknowledge the steps already taken.

COUNSELING ACTIVITY – **PRACTICING REFLECTION**

DIRECTIONS: Imagine that you are Linda and that you are talking with the dietitian. Linda says: *I'm the fat person in the room. I have always feared being fat. I thought that if I could get 'good' at dieting, then I wouldn't be fat. But I have to come to accept that I am not good at dieting. This failure, now that I am older, haunts me. I have tried so many diets that I am afraid even to tell someone I am going to try to lose weight again.*

The dietitian makes the following statements to Linda. Read each statement, and rank whether the reflection is simple (S) or complex (C). Notice how the reflection "lands," or feels, to you (Linda) when you read it. For statements that landed well, place a plus sign next to them. Statements that didn't land well get a minus sign. At the end of the list, check in with how you feel. Did these statements help you feel heard? Did the statements express empathy, prompt a conversation about understanding both sides of a problem, and support your autonomy?

- Right now, at your current size, you feel fat.
- You feel that your size is being judged by other people.
- You are feeling uncomfortable in response to this judgment.
- You would like not to be judged.
- Your hope is, by losing weight, people wouldn't judge you.
- You feel you aren't good at losing weight.
- You hope that people aren't judging you for your lack of weight loss.
- You are ashamed of this failure.
- You want people to stop judging you, so you don't tell people that you are trying to change your diet.
- You are afraid that you can't be successful unless you go on an extreme diet.
- This lack of weight loss scares you because you believe it is harming your health.

GOING DEEPER
Debriefing Practicing Reflection Statements

Now that you have practiced identifying simple and complex reflections, take a moment and list what was beneficial in doing this activity. Was it helpful to imagine being Linda? Was it helpful to just make statements instead of trying to offer solutions to the stated problem? Was it helpful to think about how these statements "land" on you the client? Was it helpful to provide both simple and complex reflections?

1. Take a moment and write down what was helpful about identifying complex and simple reflections.

2. Now list what didn't help or was confusing about the activity.

3. Stretch your skills by spending some time in reflection. Ask yourself the following four questions:

   - Have I observed the counseling technique of offering simple and complex reflections?
   - What is the benefit of simple and complex reflections? If you are not sure, where could you learn more about this Motivational Interviewing technique?
   - Have I had an opportunity to practice reflection?
   - How will I evaluate if using more reflections (either simple or complex) in my counseling session was helpful?

COUNSELING OPTIONS USING MOTIVATIONAL INTERVIEWING TO EXPLORE MINDFUL EATING

The first counseling option is OARS:

O: *Open-Ended Questions.* Ask clients about their direct experience when observing sensory information. This might sound like, "What did you notice when you checked in with your hunger?" "Describe how the meal tasted?" "What was noticeable about the experience?"

Asking the client to categorize the experience as Pleasant, Neutral, or Unpleasant can provide you with a topic to explore using Open-Ended Questions, such as, "What was it about the experience that you enjoyed?" "In what ways have you changed your eating?" "Can you give me an example of how Mindful Eating has changed your food or eating choices?"

A: *Affirm.* A simple "Thank you," "Nice," or "Well done" is often all that is needed to acknowledge the client's ability to observe sensory information. If you would like to affirm a specific behavior, it might sound like, "This is terrific that you are taking the time to cook meals you enjoy" or "Good for you! You are giving yourself permission to savor your selection." Your affirmations can also become reflections. For example, "Congratulations for checking in with your hunger before eating."

R: *Reflect.* Repeat back to the client what you heard. For example, "This is a big change, slowing down and tasting your food" or "This new behavior of checking in with your hunger before eating has been surprisingly effective."

S: *Summarize.* Focusing on Steps 1 & 2 might sound like, "Taking the time to notice your hunger has helped you enjoy eating more, because you are better able to adjust your portion size." or "You are enjoying noticing what your body is humming for and selecting these foods, instead of feeling like you should eat one specific food."

LISTENING FOR CHANGE TALK

Motivational Interviewing recommends that the counselor begin to "listen for change talk," which is defined as a desire to change, action taken to change, reasons for change, and the need for this change. The acronym for these key signs of change is DARN. Using Linda's statements, I have pulled some possible examples of DARN.

D: Desire to change: "I don't want to be afraid of being fat anymore."

A: Ability to change: The ability to not talking about weight and/or dieting.

R: Reasons for change: Fear and being afraid.

N: Need for this change: "I need to accept that I am not good at dieting."

COUNSELING ACTIVITY – DARN

DIRECTIONS: In this activity, you will explore with Linda her direct experience with the following statement: "I have tried so many diets that I am afraid even to tell someone I am going to try to lose weight again"

You ask Linda if this experience, not telling someone that she is on a diet, is Pleasant, Unsure/Neutral, or Unpleasant. If she replies:

Unpleasant: Ask open-ended questions or reflect on Linda's evaluation of not wanting to share her decision to change.

Unsure/Neutral: Ask open-ended questions or reflect on Linda's evaluation of not wanting to share her decision to change.

Pleasant: Ask open-ended questions or reflect on Linda's evaluation of not wanting to share her decision to change. Try to learn why this situation would be pleasant. You may need to guess. "You know that the judgments and suggestions of other people don't help you."

GOING DEEPER
Debriefing Listening for Change Talk

Take a moment and list what was helpful from doing this activity. Was it helpful to think up replies or statements to Linda's evaluation of the situation?

1. Take a moment and write down what you learned from the activity.
2. Now list what you would change about your counseling as a result of this activity.
3. Stretch your skills by spending some time in reflection. Ask yourself the following four questions:
   - Was it helpful to imagine how such a painful situation might be pleasant?
   - How have I observed the concept of listening to change talk presented? Where could I go for more information?
   - How can I practice listening to change talk so it feels natural and part of my normal counseling style.
   - If a reflection or statement lands wrong, how will I use the feedback so I can keep improving my counseling and continue to deepen my skills as a dietitian?

COUNSELING ACTIVITY – **SHIFTING TO ACTION TAKEN**

In this activity, you will explore with Linda her direct experience with the following statement: "Yes, I am trying to engage in self-kindness in a more consistent way." You ask Linda if this experience is Pleasant, Unsure/Neutral, or Unpleasant. She doesn't reply. You remain silent, and finally, Linda, who is looking down and talking to the floor, says: "I'm trying … to eat something at work." You guess that Linda may be struggling with self-doubt. She may not be sure if eating lunch is helping her. You need more information to help Linda learn if this experience is helping her.

In the next activity, you will have to use your imagination. Think of a client or a person you know, and imagine that this person is Linda. Your goal is to learn if eating lunch is Pleasant, Unsure/Neutral, or Unpleasant. Make statements or ask open-ended questions for each possible option, starting with:

Unpleasant: Ask open-ended questions or reflect on Linda's evaluation of eating at work. Your replies can be statements to verify that the experience is unpleasant or open-ended questions to identify whether there is any action or choice that might make the experience less unpleasant. For example, you might say, "It isn't comfortable for you to eat at work," or a question, "What foods would make eating lunch less unpleasant?"

Unsure/Neutral: Ask open-ended questions or reflect on Linda's evaluation of eating at work. Your replies can be statements to verify that the experience is Neutral, or open-ended questions to identify whether there is any action or choice that might move the experience from neutral to either Unpleasant or Pleasant. For example, you might reflect, "Eating lunch wasn't as rushed as you feared it would be." or a question, "What ideas do you have that might make eating lunch more pleasant?

Pleasant: Ask open-ended questions or reflect on Linda's evaluation of eating at work. Your replies can be statements to verify that the experience is pleasant, or open-ended questions to identify the benefit and the desire to continue this decision. For example, you might say, "It felt good to eat at lunch," or a question, "What makes this pleasant for you?"

KEEPING THE DESIRE TO CHANGE GOING

The desire to change is often not clear. Clients benefit from a chance to "walk through" a possible change. Once you hear the desire to change, you can use the following mnemonic to explore how change might come about.

COUNSELING ACTIVITY – **BECOMING ALL EARS**

Think about Linda, and imagine counseling her by:

Elaborating: Use such statements and questions as "In what ways is eating pleasant?" or "How are you going to eat lunch?" "Will you buy lunch or bring it from home?" or "Give an example of what you might eat" or "What else would make eating lunch pleasant?" "What else would make it possible for you to eat lunch?"

Affirming: Reinforce, encourage, and support the change talk. This steers a session more effectively than offering advice, because it is client-initiated.

Reflecting: Use both simple and complex reflections, keeping in mind that a complex reflection will likely provide greater clarity for the client.

Summarizing: This helps keep the change process clear and understandable.

Table 2: Using these counseling techniques together might sound like:

Mnemonic (DARN or EARS)	Client (Linda)	Response by a Counselor
Desire	"I want to eat more during the day."	
Elaborating		"In what ways?" or "How are you going to do that?" or "How will you make his happen?" or "Give an example" or "What else…?"
Ability	"I'm trying… to eat something at work."	
Elaborating or **A**ffirming		"That is great. Tell me more about this. Can you give an example of what you are eating?"
Reason	""I think eating at work will help me not overeat when I get home."	
Reflecting		"You think not eating is setting you up at night. It is creating the conditions for overeating (binge eating)."
Need for Change	"I'm afraid that my prediabetes will become diabetes if I don't change."	
Reflecting or **S**ummarizing		"Your health is changing, and you are seeing a clear connection between prediabetes and diet. You want to have more balance and a better distribution of nutrition, and you think that eating during the day will help you."

GOING DEEPER
Debriefing Shifting to Action Activities

Take a moment and list what was helpful from doing this activity.
Was it helpful to think up replies or statements to Linda's evaluation of the situation?

1. Take a moment and write down what you liked about hearing change talk.

2. How is DARN different than EARS? Write down differences between these two mnemonics.

3. Stretch your skills by spending some time in reflection. Ask yourself the following four questions:

- Where have I observed DARN and EARS being presented?
- Where can I get more support to deepen my understanding of DARN and EARS?
- Have I had an opportunity to do this in my own session? What was the outcome?
- How will I use the feedback I have received from teaching this concept to improve my counseling skills?

SOFTENING HARSH SELF-TALK

The softening of harsher self-talk might be expressed when your client begins to acknowledge effort or even progress. I find it helpful to listen for the "at-a-boy" or self-cheer such as, "I keep reminding myself to keep going" that indicates real change is happening. These small but softer statements to me indicate the arising of self-kindness. As you already learned, self-kindness and self-compassion support change.

It can be hard to train your ear to recognize change talk if you are focusing only on outcomes. A busy counseling session can require you to review some data, but focusing on weight loss, eliminating food can promote judgment. Statement from the client such as "everything is good" are not promoting change but encouraging the client to continue with the status quo. Deafness to change talk can happen if the counselor focuses, not on the client, but on a specific outcome such as weight loss or gain, improvement in blood sugar, eating meals, or not snacking.

CONNECTING

As a diabetes educator, I recognize that some appointments are full of technical information. In these education-rich sessions, it is easy to put Motivational Interviewing techniques on the shelf. When that happens, I feel so drained and empty at the end of an appointment. When I check in to my direct experience, the session is unpleasant because it lacked a sense of connection, which is something I deeply value. To help me enjoy my job, I make it a point to have some client connection time, which is what gives my job meaning and purpose. Finding balance between connection and the technical aspects of work shifts with time and experience and a healthy dose of self-compassion.

MERIT

What is "merit"? In Mindfulness, merit is a behavior or activity that, by itself, offers value despite the outcome. Examples include showing kindness toward one's self and others, meditating, pausing, being intentional, cultivating gratitude, making effort, appreciating, and becoming aware.

Merit acknowledges that, even if you practiced these behaviors every day, it is unlikely you would achieve a specific outcome (like lower cholesterol, more money, fewer wrinkles, or increased muscle tone), but your life would be enriched. The core concept of "merit" is vital in developing a Mindful Eating practice.

COUNSELING TIP

Many people are unfamiliar with the idea of merit. I ask my clients, "Are you changing? Do you think there is merit in what you are doing?" If the client believes that he is changing and that he feels he is on the "right" track, I offer him a bowl of polished stones. Clients are encouraged to take a stone as they engage in activities that represent the behaviors they are cultivating – behaviors that, by themselves, are beneficial, hence are filled with merit! When they pick out a color/shape that they like, I explain, "This is an effort stone. It takes effort to change. Let that stone remind you of your effort."

SETTING THE INTENTION

In Mindfulness, the first step of change is to set the intention, which is different from a goal. I struggle (even rebel) with our society's obsession with specific, measurable goals instead cultivating positive motivation. Goals need to be so precise with regards to human behavior that I find them to be distracting and often counterproductive. If there is too much emphasis on goals without establishing the necessary motivation to change, these very specific objectives are resented, ignored, or lost.

In your Mindful Eating practice, make the intention — a very gentle and soft desire — of bringing self-kindness/self-compassion to any and every aspect of your day. The intention need not be specific and measurable, difficult or perfunctory; it needs only to be present. Connecting with your pure desire or intention offers the necessary energy for changes. To explain the idea of intention, I would like to share a Zen story.

MERIT

Once, there was a young monk who became really interested in a particular chant. The more he chanted this ancient wisdom, the more it helped him. Time passed, and the chant became a focus of his life and study. Years passed, and he became well versed and well regarded in this passage. He learned that another monk had had this same passion for the last 60 years. He wrote to the elderly monk, who lived on a remote island, and asked whether they could meet. The older monk said he would be delighted to have a visitor. When they got together, the two monks acted like old friends as they shared their passion for this ancient chant. It was when they chanted together that the younger monk noticed that the elderly monk had been mispronouncing a few key words. The younger monk considered telling his friend, and finally gathered the courage. "You are not pronouncing these words correctly." The elderly monk was overjoyed to learn how to improve his chanting, and he thanked his friend and quickly changed. The two continued the visit in perfect harmony.

At the end the visit, as the young monk rowed his boat away, he thought about the strong and unshakable bond the two friends had formed. He was so pleased that he had been able to help his friend, to offer the proper pronunciation of those tricky words. The young monk was enjoying this daydream-like reflection when something caught his eye - a splashing on the water. He stopped rowing and tried to understand what he was seeing. The elderly monk, he realized, was running across the water, calling out his name. The elderly monk reached the boat, but he was winded, so he paused — standing there on the water. As he caught his breath, he said, "Dear friend, it seems my old mind does not remember exactly how to say the chant correctly. Would you review it with me so I say it right?" It was at this point that the younger monk realized: Sometimes, being right isn't what is important — it is our intentions that provide merit.

SEEING BARRIERS TO CHANGE

In the introduction, there is an observation that when we have support and loving people in their lives, change is easier. These supports, whether established in childhood or created in adulthood, are part of a much larger understanding of how the brain is physically wired. Dr. Daniel Siegel explains in his breakthrough book on neuropsychology, *Mindsight*[24], that creating secure attachments actually changes the structure of the brain. This sense of feeling kindness, experiencing kindness, and being with at least one person who regularly expresses kindness to a child will change how the brain is physically wired.

Unfortunately, no one has a perfect childhood. We are all left with bumps, bruises, and scars from our youth. Life is hard, and no one is spared. This fact amplifies the reason that self-kindness is so important for adults. Engaging in self-kindness rewires the brain to create a more-integrated pathway. How do we engage in self-kindness (instead of just thinking about self-kindness)? Engaging in a self-kindness meditation on a daily basis is actually rewiring the brain, helping you to make the 13-inch journey faster, easier, and more instinctively.

HOW DOES A CLIENT FEEL SELF-KINDNESS?

Now, here is a counseling tip to hold onto! Expressing empathy, evoking a conversation to understand both sides of a problem, and supporting the client's autonomy is how you, the dietitian, prepare the soil of empathy. I like to think:

> Empathy is the soil in which the seed of self-kindness can grow.

EMPATHIZING REVISITED

Take a moment and review your responses regarding three acts of self-kindness, starting with an action that takes very little effort and an action that takes more effort. Using the information that you have gained from this chapter, would you list these differently?

SELF-COMPASSION SELF-ASSESSMENT

A growing number of professionals focus on self-compassion. Dr. Kristin Neff is noted for her pioneering work on this topic. Her website offers a self-compassion assessment that is helpful for professionals (and clients). Creating Mindful Eating and nutrition programs that incorporate sufficient time to understand and explore the role of self-compassion and self-kindness can effectively counter the toxic effects of shame, discussed in Chapter 1.

To explore the concept of self-kindness and self-compassion specifically relating to body kindness, Rebecca Scritchfield, RDN, offers the book *BodyKindness*. You can learn more about her work at www.BodyKindness.com. If you are looking for more focus on food and eating, consider the work by Jean Fain, LICSW, author of *The Self-Compassion Diet: A Step-by-Step Program to Lose Weight with Loving-Kindness*. A reviewer mentioned that *The Self-Compassion Diet* does have "weight loss" in the title and expressed concerns about recommending this book. I reached out and asked Jean why she used the words "weight loss" in the title. Her thoughtful response is in the "Connecting" section.

CONNECTING

So much has changed in the last 25 years, thanks in large part to the pioneering work of Linda Bacon, who founded the Health At Every Size, or HAES movement. This organization has provided health care with some helpful guidelines that are applauded by nondiet advocates. I know Jean Fain personally and value her work. When I recently asked about "weight loss" in the title, she explained: "Back when I wrote my book (2011), I was not as familiar with the HAES research as I am now. So, in fact, it's not exactly the book I would write today. The subtitle has 'weight loss' in it, and the book talks about losing weight naturally without dieting. Over the years, I've consciously changed my language to make it weight neutral." I can empathize with Jean, being a diabetes educator who is bombarded by "scientific" evidence, journal articles, and research that talks about the importance of weight. It takes effort, care, and often many attempts to craft your HAES-friendly thoughts and views. No one is perfect, no book is perfect, and no approach is perfect, but don't let that stop you from trying!

It is my suggestion to review all books by the following HAES guidelines[25], which are that all Health At Every Size® and HAES® services/materials adhere to these basic principles:

1. **Weight Inclusivity:** Accept and respect the inherent diversity of body shapes and sizes, and reject the idealizing or pathologizing of specific weights.

2. **Health Enhancement:** Support health policies that improve and equalize access to information and services, and personal practices that improve human well-being, including attention to individual physical, economic, social, spiritual, emotional, and other needs.

3. **Respectful Care:** Acknowledge our biases, and work to end weight discrimination, weight stigma, and weight bias. Provide information and services from an understanding that socio-economic status, race, gender, sexual orientation, age, and other identities impact weight stigma, and support environments that address these inequities.

4. **Eating for Well-being:** Promote flexible, individualized eating based on hunger, satiety, nutritional needs, and pleasure, rather than any externally regulated eating plan focused on weight control.

5. **Life-Enhancing Movement:** Support physical activities that allow people of all sizes, abilities, and interests to engage in enjoyable movement, to the degree that they choose.

COUNSELING ACTIVITY – **THOUGHT COMPASS**

The Thought Compass could be a useful tool to help you better understand the concept of self-compassion and self-kindness. The Thought Compass might begin with self-kindness in the center, as depicted below, or you could map out such concepts as: the MI mnemonic EARS, HAES, exploring what merit means to you, and ideas to start your 13-inch journey. (Instructions for creating a Thought Compass are in Chapter 1.) The intention of the Thought Compass is to evoke change by calling forth your deeper wisdom.

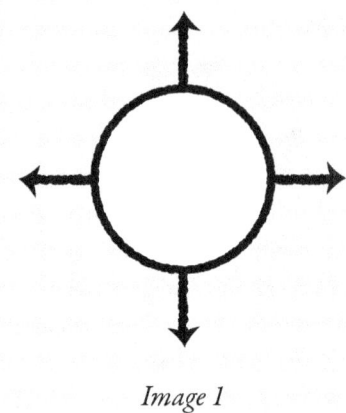

Image 1

CHAPTER SUMMARY
Defining Self-Kindness

HOORAY! Review the counseling tools you just learned.

- Self-kindness is one of the three aspects of self-compassion.

- Self-compassion counters shame, which, as you learned in Chapter 1, is a toxic emotion that stops change.

- Practicing self-kindness promotes self-compassion.

- Recognizing our common humanity promotes self-compassion.

- Becoming more mindful promotes self-compassion.

- Simple reflections help the client know that you are listening.

- Complex reflections help the client know that you understand his/her deeper emotions.

- HAES is Health At Every Size, and it offers guidelines that can help you evaluate material and move toward a more nonjudgmental stance.

OOPS! What are the struggles you might encounter?

- Self-kindness isn't a thing or a behavior, but a compassionate way of thinking.

- "There is no way to Self-Kindness, Self-Kindness is the way."

- Discussion of self-kindness may make Mindful Eating feel elusive, remote, incomprehensible to some participants.

- Self-kindness can be identified only by the client — not by the dietitian or health professional.

- Self-kindness is linked to learning and understanding what your true needs are. This can open up another area of learning for many clients, which may feel like you, the dietitian, are moving away from nutrition counseling. Referring to or working with a therapist is helpful for many clients struggling with these concepts.

- Self-criticizing is the opposite of self-kindness.

- Isolation is the opposite of common humanity.

- Overidentification is the opposite of mindfulness.

- Finding a balance among education, gathering technical information, and connecting with your client will evolve with time, experience, and practice.

TADA! Review the action steps of the chapter.

- Complete the Defining Self-Kindness activity at the beginning of the chapter. Review your answers regarding an act of self-kindness that takes little effort, more effort, and a lot of effort. Ask yourself, after reading this chapter, would you change your responses?

- Try the Self-Kindness = Equals, activity with food or eating choices.

- Write out your own intention regarding self-kindness. See how this feels different from a goal.

- Meditate on self-kindness (see Chapter 2).

- Practice self-kindness during eating and Mindful Eating activities.

- Create a formal self-reflection practice.

- Recognize self-compassion, and acknowledge this choice during a session.

- Try the self-compassion self-assessment test for personal and professional work.

- Read and review your books and print material to determine whether they meet the HAES guidelines.

- Complete a Thought Compass on the concepts of self-compassion.

SECTION TWO

Sensory/physical, Cognitive/thought, and Emotion/feelings

INTRODUCTION TO
Section Two

Section Two introduces you to the Mindful Eating Map, which is a five-step process to help an individual begin eating mindfully. In this section, you will learn to use Steps 1 and 2. In Section Three you will continue using the Mindful Eating Map and complete Steps 3-5. The purpose of the Map is to provide an overview for professionals when teaching Mindful Eating to clients. Mindful Eating is a personal journey, and the Mindful Eating Map is a guide. It is not a set of rules or requirements that are necessary for someone to eat mindfully.

HOW THE MINDFUL EATING MAP WORKS

The Mindful Eating Map is a series of five steps that provides an overview of Mindful Eating. Within each step are additional smaller steps that some individuals will like to take time to explore and understand. Each step has its own benefits, so there is no rush or need to complete all the steps in the map to eat mindfully. Step 1 focuses on nonjudgmental observation, which includes identifying three distinct experiences: sensory, thought, and emotional experience.

The ability to observe is the foundation of Mindfulness. The practice of nonjudgmental observation and is supported and deepened by regular and consistent meditation practice. When the client is ready, it is possible to move to Step 2, which is identifying and categorizing an experience as Pleasant, Neutral, or Unpleasant. The ability to apply what is observed and to categorize the information helps the client learn how to balance inner and outer information, which is a form of wisdom.

HOW SECTION TWO IS SET UP

Chapter 4 reviews the rich topic of sensory experience while eating. Here, you will identify sensory experiences, including hunger and fullness, and learn about the Six Phases of Eating. You will have a chance to use Motivational Interviewing to deepen your counseling skills and to explore the benefits of developing a reflective practice.

Chapter 5 explores how your thought experience is different than your sensory experience. Here, you will be introduced to "The Monkey Mind" and have a chance to use Motivational Interviewing techniques to help your clients observe their thought experience without getting hooked by shame, blame, or frustration.

Chapter 6 starts to make the connection between your emotional and physical experience. This is done by having you try a number of activities to make the connection. In Chapter 6, you will be introduced to techniques from Nonviolent Communications as a way to understand your needs and how your needs relate to your feelings.

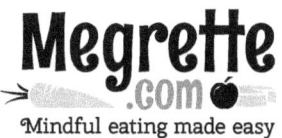

The Mindful Eating Map

By Megrette Fletcher, M.ED., RD, CDE

Step 1

1a. Stretch your ***ability to engage in non judgmental observation*** of the current situation

The current situation includes three areas of focus:

1b. Sensory experience:

taste, sight, sound, feel, hunger, fullness, satiety, wellness, illness, pain, discomfort, etc.

1c. Thought experience.

1d. Emotional experience.

Step 2.

2a. Try to ***categorize your observations***

Are they pleasant, neutral/unsure or unpleasant?

Step 3.

3a. ***Identify your personal needs*** with self-compassion.

3b. Describe the steps available to reduce the negative experience associated with your unmet needs.

3c. Dig even deeper, and add a level of self-compassion to your evaluation. What opportunities exist for you to meet your physical, emotional and social in a way that does not cause harm to yourself or others.

Step 4.

4a. *Set your* self-compassionate ***intention to reduce*** the negative experience associated with ***your unmet needs.***

4b. *Follow your intention* to reduce the negative experience associated with your unmet needs ***with self-compassion.***

Step 5.

5a. *Advocate for yourself* and all living beings ***ethically***

Mindful Eating Map is inspired by Marshall Rosenberg, CNVC.org

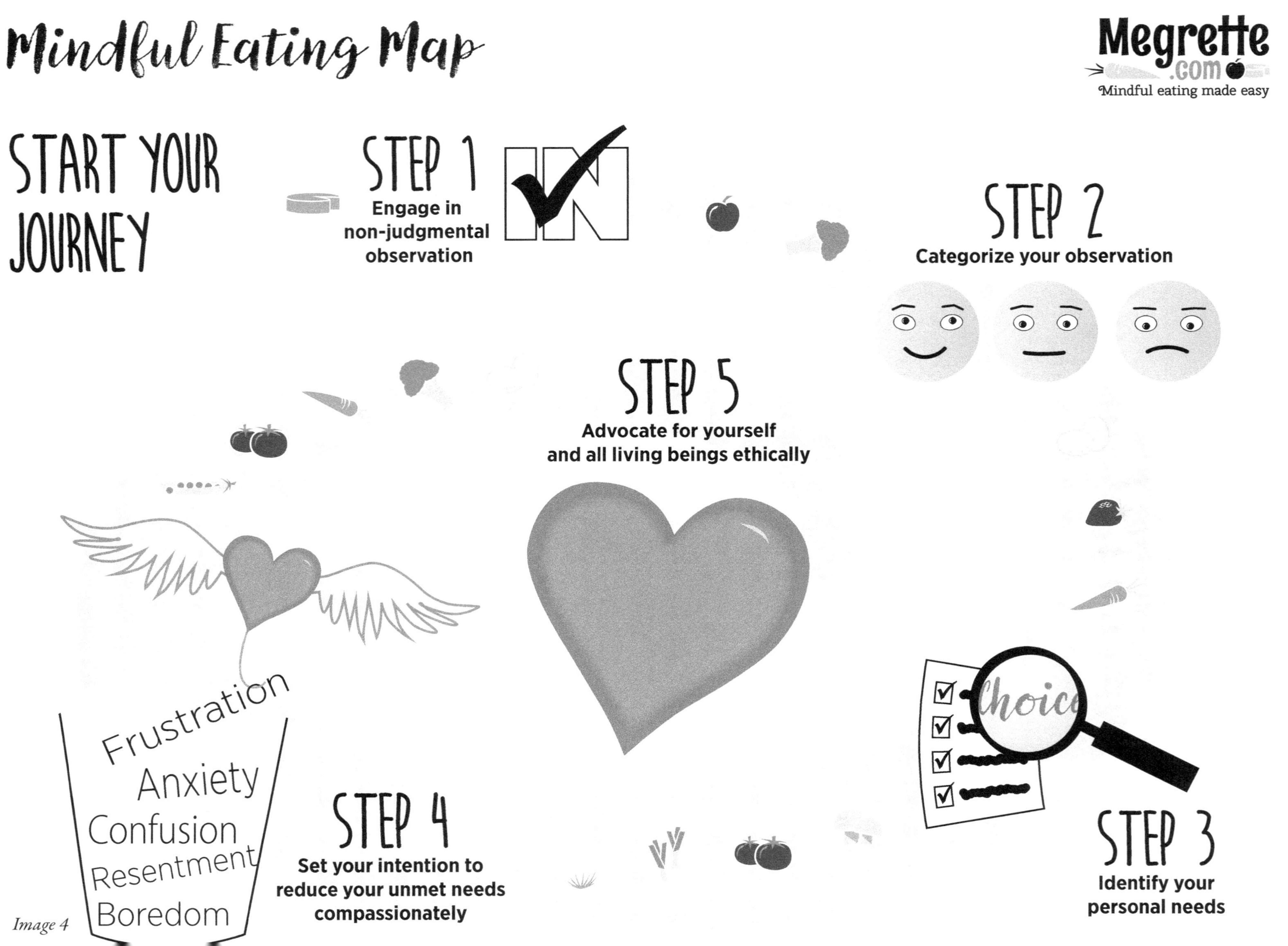

Mindful Eating Map

Megrette.com — Mindful eating made easy

START YOUR JOURNEY

STEP 1
Engage in non-judgmental observation

STEP 2
Categorize your observation

STEP 3
Identify your personal needs

STEP 4
Set your intention to reduce your unmet needs compassionately

Frustration
Anxiety
Confusion
Resentment
Boredom

STEP 5
Advocate for yourself and all living beings ethically

Image 4

EMPATHIZING - SITA

"I get into these food ruts. I think that I am adventurous, but maybe not really. I like plain food, and I do enjoy eating new things, but I typically don't like them the first time I try something. Anyway, I am back in this food rut. I can only think of 3-5 things to eat at the dining hall, and my meals are pretty boring. Can you help me?"

— Sita

CHAPTER 4
Sensory Experience While Eating

"Mindfulness transforms the mundane acts of preparing and consuming food into a memorable, multisensory experience."
— MICHELLE MAY, M.D., founder of www.AmIHungry.com and author of the book series "Eat What You Love, Love What You Eat."

Have you ever considered how your senses are engaged in eating? All five senses are receiving information when you eat. But they include more than the sight, sound, smell, taste, touch, or how something feels. They also include the sensory experience within your body, such as hunger, fullness, satiety, feelings of energy, fatigue, wellness, or illness.

The Principles of Mindful Eating says the practice uses "... all your senses in choosing to eat food that is both satisfying to you and nourishing to your body."[26] Linking The Principles of Mindful Eating to Step 1b in the Mindful Eating Map, the intention of Mindful Eating is to nonjudgmentally observe sensory experience and identify whether it is Pleasant, Neutral, or Unpleasant. Because your sensory experience is so varied and complex, there is a huge amount of information to process. Your thoughts can fib to you, saying things like, "You know what that tastes like. There is no need to waste time pausing, just eat." Over time, this becomes a habit that promotes mindless eating that might be you telling you, "Chocolate cake is good," instead of noticing the experience and asking such questions as, "Is *this* chocolate cake good? Would chocolate cake taste good to me now, at this moment?"

In this chapter, you are going to explore how to pause and "check in" to observe (nonjudgmentally) your sensory experiences and to let this guide you in determining whether the experience is Pleasant, Neutral, or Unpleasant. You will also unpack the concept of habitual reactions that prevent you from observing sensory experience. You will explore the Six Phases of Eating as a tool to "check in" to sensory experience.

REFLECTING – EXPLORING SENSORY EXPERIENCE

Jan Chozen Bays, MD, explains in her book *Mindful Eating: A Guide to Rediscovering a Healthy and Joyful Relationship With Food*[27]: "Mindful Eating is an experience that engages all parts of us — our body, our heart, our mind — in choosing, preparing, and eating food. Mindful Eating involves all the senses. It immerses us in the color, texture, scents, tastes, and even sounds of drinking and eating. It allows us to be curious and even playful as we investigate our responses to food and our inner cues to hunger and satisfaction." In this description of Mindful Eating, you can see that the beginning of eating the meal is a playground of distractions. Every sensory receptor is engaged, and in a moment, you are transported to a whole new world of experience.

Your sensory experience is a big part of the internal information that needs to be processed when making a food choice.

It is considered internal because no one but you knows if you are hungry or full, or like or dislike food — unless you tell them. Your sensory information can also guide your food and eating choices to nourish your body. Observe what your body is wanting. Is it crunch or sweet, the chew of protein or a soft roll? Learning to listen to these internal requests will aid in the food-selection process.

Observing your sensory experience while eating can also guide your decision to continue or to stop eating, based on your level of fullness and growing sense of satiety. It is easy to see that your sensory information is an important part of the eating experience, not just to enjoy eating, but also to assist you in meeting nutrient and energy needs.

COUNSELING ACTIVITY – **THE FOOD HOOK**

To begin, engage in an observation activity that should take less than 60 seconds and that connects you with your sensory experiences. These observations are called scans. They begin with your direct sensory experience and can be specific — notice hunger or fullness or a general discomfort or pleasure. Before eating, noticing your sensory experience nonjudgmentally is the first part of a two-part process. The second part is to notice your sensory experience *while* eating. This is much more challenging because your sensory experiences are already engaged by the mere presence of food. This means the hook of taste, smell, texture, or sound might have grabbed your mind and is making it really, really, really hard to remain a nonjudgmental observer. See for yourself.

Part 1

Sit comfortably, letting your focus soften before you, or close your eyes if that is more comfortable. Breathe in deeply, then slowly exhale. Repeat this three times. Now, on the fourth breath, notice how the air feels moving into your nose. Notice the air as it leaves your nose or mouth. How would you describe this experience? Is it Pleasant, Neutral, or Unpleasant? With your next breath, notice your chest filling with air. Notice how it rises and falls as the air moves in and out of the chest. Now observe your sense of hunger. Is it Pleasant, Neutral, or Unpleasant? Take three deep breaths as you did in the beginning, and open your eyes. Use *Image 5*, the Three Faces, to help you identify your direct experience.

Image 5

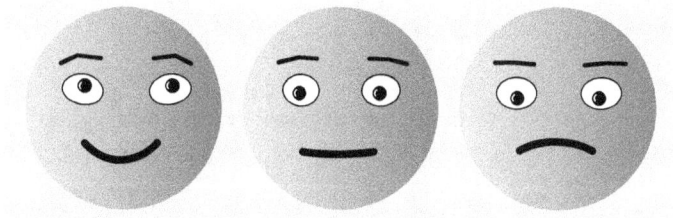

Part 2: Get up and get a snack or something to eat. Return to your seat.

Sit comfortably, holding the food on a plate or towel. Focus on the food before you, or close your eyes if that is more comfortable. Breathe in and out. Repeat this three times and on the fourth breath, notice your sensory experience. Notice the air as it leaves your nose or mouth. Can you smell the food? With your next breath, notice your chest filling with air. Notice how it rises and falls as the air moves in and out of the chest. Now observe your sense of hunger. Is it Pleasant, Neutral, or Unpleasant? Take three deep breaths as you did in the beginning, and open your eyes. Observe your sensory experience, specifically your sense of hunger. Was there a difference between noticing your hunger when food was present? Describe if this difference was Pleasant, Neutral, or Unpleasant. Use Image 1 to help you identify your direct experience.

EMPATHIZING: SENSORY EXPERIENCE

If you completed the activity of observing your sensory experience while food was present, you likely noticed how difficult it was to observe your senses and not get hooked by the craving and desire for food. Just having an enjoyable food in proximity can start the all-too-familiar craving cycle that seems to play in your head.

People frequently ask me, "How do I stop craving? How do I stop having these thoughts?" My response is: You don't stop craving or desire. You can learn to tolerate them, even welcome them to a meal. This may seem like a dream, or a far-fetched goal that you might reach for, until you begin to understand that cravings and desire are temporary experiences. Clients will tell me, "I always crave [X]." My response is to smile because I know either that this statement is true and we can work on enjoying such a persistent experience or that this statement isn't 100% true, but is the client's mind creating this story, so the client believes it to be true.

CRAVINGS ARE NOT BAD

The tendency to label everything as "good" or "bad" is a story that the busy, rushing mind likes to tell. The story might start like this: "It is faster to stick a 'black or white,' 'good or bad' label on something than it is to take the time to observe and evaluate." Sound familiar? Initially, these stories are trying to make a difficult situation easier, but as habits go, the mind thinks, "Well, it worked here. Let's do that again!" This story starts getting repeated until everything has a label. Unfortunately, labeling something "good" or "bad" is a form of judgment that only energizes your craving experience. You may find yourself spending time and energy worrying, fearing, avoiding, and wrestling with a craving, instead of choosing to experience it.

CONNECTING

Many years ago, I had the opportunity to listen to His Holiness the Dalai Lama speak. He offered the audience a question that I would like to share with you.

If you had everything you could ever craved, would you stop craving?

The question changed my mind, because, until that moment, I thought I could free myself of craving. What I realized is that I can't stop cravings from arising. I almost panicked, until His Holiness explained that cravings are part of the human condition. Phew, I am normal, and when I am hooked by a juicy craving, I return to this reassuring memory. Shifting my thinking from trying to stop craving to accepting craving created a new sense of space. In this space, I connected to the common humanity and decrease sense of isolation. This allowed me to discover a choice I didn't know existed.

Instead of applying effort and energy, refocus on your sensory experience. Pause and check in with your senses. As you pause, become clear with what is actually present vs. what fleeting thought or desire is popping up. Many people are afraid to do this because, they worry, smelling or tasting something yummy will only make the craving worse. If this concern is present, see whether there is another option. Take a moment and observe the possibilities.

COUNSELING ACTIVITY – THOUGHT COMPASS ON SENSORY EXPERIENCE

To do this, place "my cravings" in the center of the Thought Compass diagram, and explore all the ideas and options you want to try. Many people will modify the environment, for example, by purchasing a small bag of chips instead of a family-size bag; eating with a supportive person or group; eating when physical hunger is neutral or comfortable, instead of when hunger is large and uncomfortable. These examples are often provided in magazines and life-hack tips on social media posts. Susan Albers, PsyD, and author of many Mindful Eating books, including *50 Ways to Soothe Yourself Without Food*[28], provides many examples of how to make a craving more tolerable.

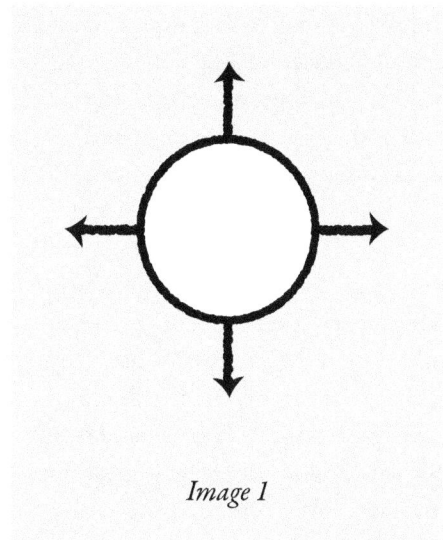

Image 1

WHAT IS PHYSICAL HUNGER?

How is physical hunger different from other types of hunger? First, physical hunger builds slowly. It doesn't just "pop" into your head. Physical hunger typically happens a few hours after your last meal. It will have more than one symptom that is felt in the lower part of the body, typically in the small V-shaped space between your ribs and belly button.

Quick Summary: Physical hunger is a slow-building sensation that has multiple cues and is felt typically in the upper abdominal area.

Is it hard for you to determine whether you are hungry or full? If you struggle with this, learning about hunger and fullness may feel strange, foreign, even unnecessary. What I can share is that the growing amount of research has confirmed that avoiding, ignoring, or denying hunger via restrictive eating – a.k.a. dieting — doesn't work. In fact, the 2016 American Academy of Pediatrics guidelines identified dieting as one of the five factors associated with obesity and eating disorders.

> "Dieting (defined as caloric restriction with the goal of weight loss) is a risk factor for both obesity and eating disorders. One study found that teens who diet are two to three times more likely to become overweight and one and a half times more likely to develop binge-eating disorder than teens who don't diet. Dieting has emerged as the most important predictor to developing an eating disorder. One study showed that teens who severely restricted their caloric intake and skipped meals were 18 times more likely to develop an eating disorder than nondieters; more moderate dieters were five times more likely to develop an eating disorder.[30]"

This statement is a powerful reminder that dieting is how you learn to have disordered and disconnected eating habits. As you start your journey in Mindful Eating, begin by "checking in." Observe your experience with hunger, and notice the sensation of blood-sugar shift, rumblings, and grumblings in your stomach. As you check in, Mindful Eating asks that you understand there isn't a specific experience you are trying to have or a feeling that is "right" or a sign of hunger that is "good." In Mindful Eating, we shift our thinking from "Good and Bad" to simple curiosity. Questions such as, "What is my experience?" "Is this experience Pleasant, Neutral, Unpleasant?" "What would help me ease this level of hunger?" are great ways to learn more about your food and eating choices. Curiosity about the sensations of hunger and fullness can start an internal conversation, increase the variety of your food eat, and create body trust. Also, by shifting to a curious, nonjudgmental stance, you are learning from both the pleasant and unpleasant experiences with food and eating. This is a great way of discovering there are no "Bad" opportunities to learn, just some you enjoy more!

Remember that the experience of physical hunger is a group of signals. Think of hunger as a detective game in which there are three or four clues, and your job is to determine whether it is physical hunger or something else, such as hunger influenced by your mood, emotions, or proximity to food. Here are 14 signs that are associated with hunger: pangs, growling, grumbling, emptiness, gnawing, queasy feeling, tired, low energy, weak, irritability, mild headache, difficulty concentrating, thinking, or making decisions. Are any present? Your internal conversation might sound like:

- "When was the last time I ate?"
- "What did I have?"
- "Could this be hunger?"
- "Describe the feeling in my stomach."
- "Am I feeling tired?"
- "Do I have a headache?"
- "Is there a touch of irritability in my voice?"
- "Could this be hunger? Or is this just a difficult situation?"

Checking in is important because eating *only fixes hunger, nothing more*. Eating when you are not physically hungry does not give you energy, a sense of calm, or a sense of health. It doesn't make a difficult situation easy. It doesn't make fatigue from a bad night's sleep go away. Eating when you are not physically hungry is using food as a way to cope, which offers a temporary solution, but once the food is gone, you need either a new way to cope or more food.

When the body does not need more energy, and you overfill it with energy from food (that is, eating when you are not physically hungry), your body is forced to deal with something it doesn't need. Think of it like this: Eating when you are not hungry is the same as trying to put 20 gallons of gas in your car when you have a 15-gallon tank. That doesn't help the car or make it go farther. It just causes a mess for the car and distress for you.

What to do? Start by exploring your hunger/fullness experience. Any hunger/fullness scale can help you learn to identify your physical hunger. However, the following hunger/fullness scale that incorporates the concepts of Uncomfortable (in red), Comfortable (in blue), and Neutral (in green) is something I found helpful when teaching this concept. This full-color handout is available for download at www.mindfuleatingforkids.com.

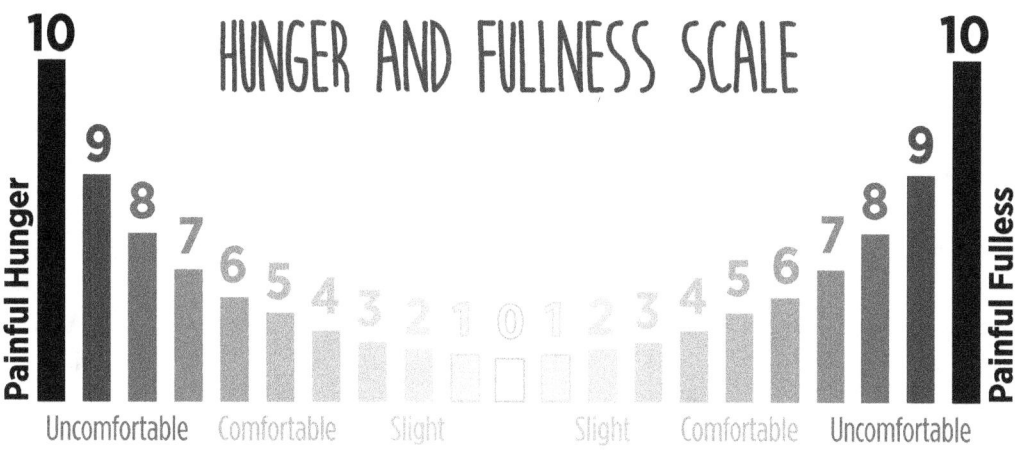

Image 6

The ability to connect your direct experience with Pleasant, Neutral, or Unpleasant is an essential part of your Mindful Eating journey. *Image 6*, the bar chart version of the Hunger and Fullness Scale, shows each experience is greatest at level 10. Think of this like a volume knob. Ten is the loudest, and when you eat, the sound becomes softer until the sound of hunger is silent.

At this point, hunger is no longer present. This is an important experience: If you keep turning the knob, you are getting a different sound, and it is telling you about a different signal. The new signal is fullness, and if you listen, you are now hearing how full you are. Fullness will become louder and louder until it is Uncomfortable.

An important teaching point is this: You don't have to check in with hunger or fullness. You don't have to eat when you are hungry and stop when you are full. You don't have to wait until you are a specific number on the Hunger and Fullness Scale. These are just another form of control and restriction. The reason Mindful Eating asks you to check in with your hunger and fullness is to help you enjoy eating. When you connect with the reason you are eating — to enjoy the experience — the shoulds, have-tos, and musts drop away. Let enjoyment join the eating party! If you are working with younger children, *Image 7*, The Hunger and Fullness Peas, is a Hunger and Fullness Scale that provides an understandable illustration of this concept for children. This is also available in full color at www.mindfuleatingforkids.com.

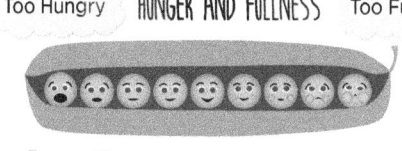

Image 7

COUNSELING ACTIVITY – HUNGER AND FULLNESS

Using the above Hunger and Fullness Scale, draw a smiley face that would indicate which eating experience is Pleasant, which is Neutral, and which is Unpleasant. Using a smiley face, ask yourself, "What is my experience when I under- or overeat?" If you are working with a client, continue to have him check in with his direct experience with food and eating. If a client indicates that an experience is Pleasant, learn what makes it pleasant. Affirm this experience, "Eating is pleasant," and compare it with other desires and needs. For example, "Eating when I was hungry felt better than eating when I was starving."

Open-Ended Question: "How did eating at this level of hunger change your energy level?" or "Did eating at this level of hunger change how much you ate at the meal?"

SIX PHASES OF EATING

Before The Center for Mindful Eating was established, very little information was available about Mindful Eating. This lack of information prompted Fred Burggraf and me to write *Discover Mindful Eating*. After creating 51 handouts about Mindful Eating, we had a lot of discussion about how to organize them. We both struggled to create a logical way to start teaching Mindful Eating. Both Fred and I could see that, although eating had been traditionally regarded as a single activity, the process was far more complex than that! After many conversations, we had a breakthrough and — Voilà! — The Six Phases of Eating. In the book *Discover Mindful Eating*, my co-author and I explain that the act of eating isn't one step, but six. *Image 8* provides a graphical representation of the Six Phases of Eating.

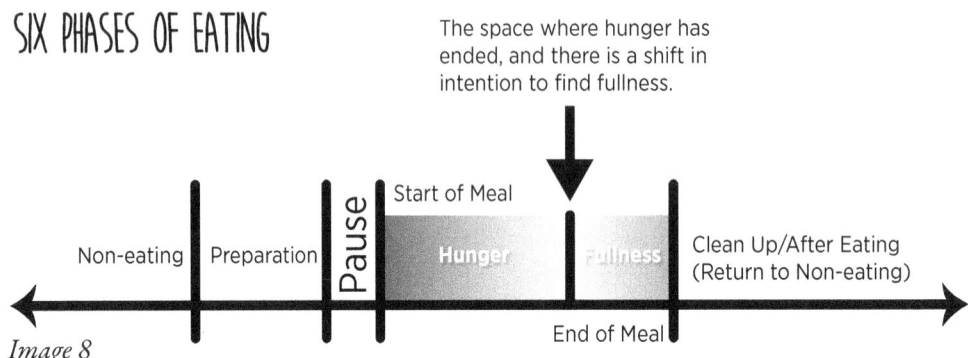

Image 8

UNDERSTANDING THE SIX PHASES

1. **Non-eating.** In this phase, a person would not eat. There is no physical sense of hunger present. This would be represented by a by a hunger/fullness rating of 0. If hunger were present, the individual would move to the preparation phase.

2. **Preparation.** This phase involves the selecting of what to eat. It is a daunting task. As Brian Wansink's research showed in the book *Mindless Eating*[29], each of us makes more than 200 daily decisions surrounding food! If hunger is present, there may be a desire to snack before a meal. However, hunger may not always be present — for example, when food shopping for the week. Many people like engaging in meal preparation when hunger is slight or not present, because they find they are better able to make choices that are balanced and that nourish the body.

3. **Pause.** This phase happens before eating. It is connected with your physical sense of hunger, but the pause does more. It connects you with your intention for self-kindness — or at least to not harm yourself.

4. **Eating.** Awareness of your level of hunger (or fullness) is present. While eating, notice your direct sensory experience: sight, sound, smell, taste, touch, or how something feels. Keep in mind that your sensory experience also involves your body, such as hunger, fullness, satiety, feelings of energy, fatigue, wellness, or illness.

5. **End of meal.** In this phase, you are aware that your physical hunger has ended and that fullness has started to emerge. If you keep eating, fullness will increase from the level of 1 (slight) to 4-6 (comfortable). If you continue eating, the level will increase past comfort to an uncomfortable level 7+.

6. ***Clean up and a return to non-eating.*** In this phase, you have some level of fullness, which is likely why you stopped eating. However, it is also likely you are still surrounded by sensory temptation. This makes the Clean-Up Phase different from the Non-Eating Phase because it requires an additional awareness of the environmental cues that may prompt a person to keep eating, which is called Mindless Eating.

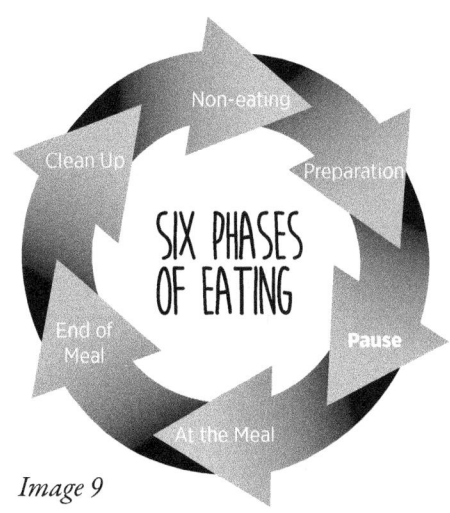

Image 9

Many people are unaware that the Six Phases of Eating are not necessarily linear, as presented in *Image 8*, but are cyclical, as depicted in the *Image 9*, The Six Phases of Eating Cycle

GOING DEEPER
Balancing Sensory Information with Self-Kindness

If you eat when you are comfortably hungry and stop when you are comfortably full, you might notice that eating is enjoyable. You may not do this 100% of the time because overeating or undereating at times might also be enjoyable. Setting the intention, however, to make eating an enjoyable experience starts the process of your balancing sensory information with self-kindness. As you learned in Chapter 3, self-kindness is part of the larger concept of self-compassion. In the Mindful Eating Map, Step 3c asks: "What opportunities exist for you to meet your physical, emotional, and social needs in a way that does not cause distress or harm to yourself or others?"

This means that if overeating or undereating is causing harm, you may choose to take steps to shift your behaviors — not to achieve an outcome like weight loss or lower cholesterol, but to ease the discomfort caused by your unpleasant sensory experiences.

Awareness of your sensory experiences includes sight, sound, smell, taste, touch, or how something feels, as well as the sense experiences within our bodies, such as hunger, fullness, satiety, feelings of energy, fatigue, comfort, discomfort, wellness, or illness. You may discover that few foods or eating situations can meet all of your sensory desires. Therefore, you may direct your intention to a specific awareness, for example, the look of food or the level of satiety you feel. Maybe it is a taste, like something tart, or just the desire to crunch on something. You may modify your choices to increase energy or a sense of wellness. With awareness, you are likely to discover the huge amount of flexibility, choice, and freedom that comes when you eat mindfully. With practice, tiny shifts to make a meal or food choice more pleasant become easier and almost unconscious.

As Mindful Eating moves from your head to heart, you may hear yourself saying, "I am not eating slower because I should, or it will help me lose weight. I am eating slower so I can enjoy my meal, my choice, the bite, and savor each mouthful of food."

BECKONING OR HUMMING

Being aware of your direct sensory experience can help you distinguish whether food is "beckoning" — or motioning you to come. Beckoning represents your food desires in a sweet, simple way that I find easier to understand than craving, which can have a negative connotation.

Foods that are "Humming" fill you with a sense of energy and enjoyment that vibrates with joy. Using myself as an example, peanut butter is food that I typically Hum for. More often than not, when I eat peanut butter; I feel my whole body humming with joy.

COUNSELING ACTIVITY – **TRY BECKONING OR HUMMING**

Pause. Using all your senses, ask yourself whether there is food available that will help your body hum. Is there food available that beckons to you?

LISTENING FOR CHANGE TALK

There is a natural assumption that the desire to change some aspect of the sensory experience is brought about by unpleasant experiences. For example, imagine you ate something and thought, "This is really gross!" You might assume that would make you want to change. But this is not necessarily true. Some sensory experiences feel gross simply because they are new or a shock to the taste buds. Many people are willing to keep eating a food despite its taste.

Understanding the unspoken desire requires good counseling and some detective work. I have found the Discover, Explore, Play, and Challenge exercise helpful in uncovering unspoken desires lurking inside.

▶ ***Discover.*** What you actually desire often requires reflection. There are many different ways to connect with your unspoken desire. Set aside time for some type of daily contemplative practice. Reflective techniques described in this book so far include meditation and Thought Compass. If you are looking to explore other contemplative techniques, consider using The Tree of Contemplative Practices[31]. Daily reflection can help you start the process of listening to your own thoughts, hopes, wishes, and needs, helping you become clear on what you truly desire.

▶ Once you discover what you want, ***Explore*** your options. For example, say you discovered that you are hungry at lunch, but that your typical lunch wasn't really filling you up. You may want to find out what other lunch options are available or even possible for you. You decide on having soup for lunch, but there are a lot of options available that you could play with.

▶ This is where ***Play*** comes in. Trying different soup options can be fun. You may go on Pinterest or Facebook, buy some cookbooks, or talk with friends about their favorites — all part of the Play phase.

▶ ***Challenge***, the last phase, is when you focus on your plan. In this phase, you are challenging yourself to change, and maybe stick to your soup and salad plan for the next week and then re-evaluate your options.

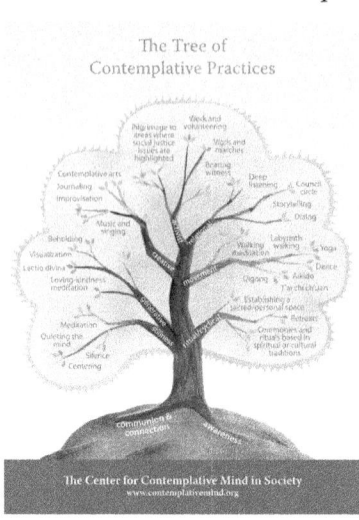

Graphic 1

In a more complex example, say you *discover* you want to stop dieting (restrictive eating). **Explore** what that desire really means. Reflect on how you feel when you hear restrictive messages in society, in health care, or from friends.

As you explore these messages, **play** with alternatives, conversation comebacks, and other ways to meet your need to move away from restrictive eating. Finally, **challenge** yourself and your friends to stop talking about the latest diet or weight-loss attempt.

COUNSELING ACTIVITY – DISCOVER, EXPLORE, PLAY, AND CHALLENGE

Read the section below, which is part of a counseling session with Sita.

> *I'm not sure what I want. I think that is the hardest part of changing your diet. Meal planning is new to me. I come up with five or so recipes that they serve in the dining hall, and in a few days, I am in a rut. My friend who is vegan suggested that we get each other lunch. We would put our plates in the center of the table and each take from the bounty that we each got. That was fun! I loved doing that. I tried a lot of new foods that way, and we would laugh so much!*

DIRECTIONS: Imagine you wrote Discover, Explore, Play, and Challenge on a piece of paper and handed it to Sita. You say, "Sita, would you pick one of these words to best describe the phase you are in?" What is Sita's desire?

Using your own counseling experience, what open-ended question could you ask to explore Sita's unspoken desire?

GOING DEEPER
Debriefing Desire

1. Take a moment and write down what you liked about using Discover, Explore, Play, and Challenge to reveal a client's unspoken desire.

2. What didn't you like about the activity? How would you change it to better meet your needs?

3. Stretch your skills by spending some time in reflection. Ask yourself the following four questions:

- How can I make the change process fun and engaging?
- How can I convey this concept using my own words and experiences?
- Have I had an opportunity to teach the science of change to my clients?
- After I try something new at a session, class, or group, how will I use the feedback I have received?

DARN (REVISITED) — MOTIVATIONAL INTERVIEWING MNEMONIC FOR HEARING CHANGE TALK

Motivational Interviewing has the mnemonic DARN. Keep this in mind when listening for change talk. Once a person has started the change process, the "A" in DARN can shift from Ability to Action.

D: *Desire.* The willingness to change some aspect of the sensory experience.

A: *Action.* Steps taken to change some aspect of the sensory experience, such as trying new foods, new tastes, new ways of preparing, or returning to behaviors and strategies that were effective. For example, adding crunch to yogurt really helped you enjoy eating it.

R: *Reflection.* Understanding whether an experience was Pleasant, Neutral, or Unpleasant can help you understand the reason for change. Maybe having an OK-tasting food that makes you feel great is enough to make a neutral experience become pleasant. Maybe not feeling hungry in an hour makes the eating pleasant. The reason you change what you are eating is so complex that it is OK to give yourself time and space to really think about it.

N: *Need.* In the Mindful Eating Map, this is step 3, which you will learn more about later. For now, I will say that understanding and expressing your needs is not an easy task. Getting your needs met is a lifelong process — not to mention that your needs change all the time! Deep breath, continue to practice steps 1 and 2 to help complete step 3.

CHAPTER SUMMARY
Sensory Experience While Eating

HOORAY! Review the counseling tools you just learned.

Tools to assist the client are:

- Teaching models for checking in with your sensory experience:
- The Hunger and Fullness Rating Scale
- The Six Phases of Eating

Concepts presented are:

- Beckoning and Humming, which can be a gentle way of understanding craving vs. self-care food choices.
- Exploring desire by using the Discover, Explore, Play, and Challenge format.
- Listening for desire, using Motivational Interviewing's DARN mnemonic.

OOPS! Review the struggles you might encounter.

- There are many types of sensory information to focus on.
- Sensory information can "hook" your mind and create distracting thoughts.
- People develop habitual reactions to situations as a way to save time. These reactions or decisions become invisible to us over time. It can be challenging to guide a client to become aware of them.
- Some people think there is a "right" hunger level to determine when to eat, or a correct fullness to stop eating. This is another form of restrictive eating. The reason to start or stop eating is created by connecting to awareness of pleasure and to an emerging sense of self-kindness.

TADA! Review the action steps of the chapter.

- Practice strengthening your skill of nonjudgmental observation of the current situation.
- Stretch this skill to include sensory experience: taste, sight, sound, feel, hunger, fullness, satiety, etc.
- Identify your sensory experience as Pleasant, Neutral, or Unpleasant.
- Create a Thought Compass of what you have learned from this chapter.

EMPATHIZING – SITA

"I am in my dorm room, and I am really dreading the dining hall. I miss 'my' food, you know the soups that my mom made. I am eating crap, and it is so frustrating to me. I don't feel good after I eat, but I also can't seem to figure out what to have. The plates are so small, and the lines are so long. If I try something that I don't like, I don't seem to have time to get something different. I know that they can make me something special, but that is such a pain. I really wish it was easier to eat a vegan diet."

— Sita

CHAPTER 5
Thought Experience

"As you are eating, become aware of the thoughts flying through your head — notice them, but do not indulge them or give in to them. Simply let them rise and fall without becoming ensnared by them."
— REBECCA GLADDING, MD, "The Perils of Multitasking," Food for Thought

So far, you have learned that Mindful Eating is the ability to observe nonjudgmentally the sensory information that comes from the five senses — sight, sound, smell, taste, touch, or how something feels – as well as the sense experience within our bodies, such as hunger, fullness, satiety, feelings of energy, fatigue, wellness, or illness. We are going to expand this skill of observing sensory information to include your thoughts. A person's thoughts are like the clouds that cover the sky. In a blink of the eye, we forget that behind the clouds is the sky, because when we look up, we see just the clouds, and we wonder if those clouds mean rain. Our thoughts take our mind in many directions. This fickle nature of the mind, which is to move from one distraction to another, is one of the reasons Mindfulness and Mindful Eating offer so many other benefits, from reducing stress and improving memory to changing how the brain works.

THE PROBLEM WITH THOUGHTS

One problem is we don't notice that we are thinking. Sensory information is easier to spot because you can look, smell, taste, touch, etc., by directing your attention to one of your senses. Sure, it takes some practice, but it is pretty clear what to do.

Thoughts, on the other hand, lack a way to notice them. Adding to the challenge is that your experiences are also influenced by your emotions, your past, and your present. In short, your thoughts are tangled up in your needs, feelings, and sensory experience.

The ability to untangle your thoughts from your feelings and sensory experience is almost inhuman. Mere mortals like you and me are not meant to be perfect at this. We are meant to try. Which is why the word "practice" is emphasized. Mindfulness helps you untangle your thoughts from your feelings by developing the ability to observe your thoughts. In other words, Mindfulness practice requires you to notice you are thinking, nothing more. It does not ask you to identify, understand, explain, or communicate what you are thinking.

WHY OBSERVE YOUR THOUGHTS?

Thinking can pull you away from the present moment. Thinking is also tangled up in your feelings, your sensory experience, your past, present, and future. It is easy to connect with your chattery mind and lose focus. The chatty mind is sometimes called a Monkey Mind, because, like a monkey, thoughts jump from idea to idea, grabbing at anything they can hold on to, screeching and chattering away.

It is an amazing ability to notice you are thinking, to pause and observe that you are not attending to the task at hand, for example, preparing dinner, but remembering something that happened last week at work that continues to bother you. This information provides you with a choice.

Return to the task of preparing dinner, or decide to understand what is happening at work. You might think, Why not do both? When you try to divide your attention, your chattery mind gets louder. More and more thoughts flood your mind, pulling it in many more directions. This ping-ponging from one idea to another can be stressful, and it seems to obscure our memories. You "forget" what you were doing, lose track of where you were, or get confused about the next step. If you have been experiencing any of these symptoms, try mindfully focusing on the task at hand, without doing anything else. One suggestion on how to do this is to review Chapter 2, and the 3D meditation. This brief meditation can help re-focus the mind.

THE BENEFIT OF OBSERVATION

You may have forgotten that the first step of the scientific method is observation. Observing your thoughts, instead of focusing on what you are thinking about, is the initial step of Mindfulness and Mindful Eating. As you observe your thoughts, you will likely notice that some feelings will arise. This is normal and expected. Watch the feelings, and let them pass by. You will notice that your feelings seem to bubble up the more you observe. They come, they go, they float on by and rise high up into the sky. In a short time, patterns emerge. The next step is to decide whether your thoughts are Pleasant, Neutral, or Unpleasant. As you observe your thoughts, you are stopping your brain from telling stories. Dan Siegel of the Mindsight Institute says, "The mind is constantly creating a coherent narrative."[32] This is a nice way of saying that, unless you are observing your thoughts, you are likely getting pulled into the story. Now, many people wonder, "What is so bad with thinking about things?" Nothing is bad about it, but very quickly, your thoughts become juicy, interesting, ego-stroking stories that pull you out of your observer's chair and into the drama that is happening in your head. Brené Brown, PhD, author and shame researcher, offers a clever way to remember you are telling stories. In her book *Raising Strong*[33] she suggests starting a comment with the reminder, "The story that I am telling myself is..."

Allowing yourself to remember that the mind tells stories offers you a choice. It removes you from the chatter and lets you watch the story instead of getting sucked into the action. Some stories are new, and it makes sense that you get drawn into them. However, most stories are not new. In fact, they seem to repeat day after day. The ability to observe these stories help you recognize a repeating pattern.

COUNSELING ACTIVITY – **THE PLAYBILL**

The purpose of this exercise is to practice observing thoughts. One way to do this is to summarize what an imaginary "performance" is about. You will use Sita's statement.

DIRECTIONS: Read the following dialog and complete the "Playbill" below.

Yesterday in the dining hall, there was nothing to eat. I mean, nothing. I had to ask them to make me a tofu stir fry. It was fine, but by the time I got my meal, all of my friends were done eating. I was struggling because I really like this meal, and I almost never get it. It is really delicious, and they cook the tofu with a sauce that I like. I love all the colors, and I guess it reminds me of home. It is something I like to savor. My friends were staring at me with that "hurry up" look. I told them, "Go ahead," so they left. I was all alone in the dining room, and I felt like such an outcast.

Describe what The Play is about: Sita finding vegan dining options at college.

Describe what the struggle is: The conflict that Sita feels about becoming vegan, which requires special food and often more preparation time, and about fitting in with her college friends.

List the sensory experience described: Savor, taste, color.

Reflect the story back to the client: You were disappointed that your friends wouldn't wait for you at dinner. You were excited to have a meal you really liked the taste of, but you didn't enjoy eating it because you were all alone.

DIRECTIONS: Read the following dialog and complete the "Playbill" below.

Yesterday at the dining hall, there were no bowls, so I couldn't make my high-protein oatmeal. I just couldn't stomach eating the eggs — yuck! I walked around and decided to have some fruit. I knew I was more hungry than that, but I couldn't think of what else to have.

Describe what The Play is about:

Describe what the struggle is:

List the sensory experience described:

Reflect the story back to the client:

GOING DEEPER
Debriefing The Playbill Activity

1. Take a moment and write down what you liked about the Playbill activity.

2. What didn't you like about the activity? How would you change it to better meet your needs?

3. Stretch your skills by spending some time in reflection. Ask yourself the following two questions:

- How have I observed the concept of the mind telling stories? Think about the "client's story" to identify how this can help me create simple or complex reflections to share during a session.

- How can I convey this concept using my own words and experiences?

COUNSELING ACTIVITY – **COUNTERING THOUGHT STORIES**

Read the statements below.

- *I can't remember to eat breakfast in the morning.*
- *There are never any vegan meals*
- *I have never liked soy products, like the fake meat. To me it is gross. I don't want to eat animals, and I don't want to eat vegetables that are made to look like meat either.*
- *I am always disappointed with my options. For example, today there were two vegetarian options. One was a vegetable scramble with soy meat, and the other was pasta with cheese. Neither of these options appealed to me.*

Using Brown's suggestion, recast the above sentences:

- *The story that I am telling myself is I can't remember to eat breakfast in the morning.*
- *The story that I am telling myself is there are never any vegan meals.*
- *The story that I am telling myself is I have never liked soy products like the fake meat.*
- *The story that I am telling myself is I am always disappointed with my options.*

Did anything shift when you did this? Take a moment and write down what you noticed.

_____
_____
_____
_____

HOW MINDFULNESS CAN HELP

Mindfulness can help in two ways. First, is the story fiction or nonfiction? If even a part of this story is fiction, pause and ask, "Why would I tell a story that wasn't 100% true?" (HINT: Because that is what our minds do — they like to fib or tell juicy stories!)

GOING DEEPER
Debriefing Countering Stories Activity

1. Take a moment and write down what you liked about the Countering Stories activity.
2. What didn't you like about the activity? How would you change it to better meet your needs?
3. Stretch your skills by spending some time in reflection. Ask yourself the following three questions:

- How have I observed this concept being presented? Am I interested in reading Brené Brown's book *Rising Strong*?
- How can I convey this concept using my own words and experiences?

THE TIME MACHINE

Your thoughts fuel your story, which you repeat over and over again. For example, you smell something that reminds you of your childhood, a time when you wanted to buy a cinnamon roll, but you couldn't. Maybe the thought in your head right now is a bit complex and hard to sort out, yet the urge is clear, and it is swirling around the idea to purchase and eat a cinnamon roll.

In the above example, the smell of cinnamon prompted you stepped into a Time Machine. You can see the how the time machine of your thoughts works. You smelled something (sensory experience), and in an instant, you were transported back to childhood. It doesn't matter that your childhood was decades ago. The time machine of the mind will take you into a story from your past better than a blockbuster Hollywood movie! Your thoughts can transport you into the future or past, or to random fantasy lands. The idea of having a time machine almost sounds enjoyable until you realize that, if your mind is ping-ponging from one thought to another, it might not feel so relaxed. In fact, you might feel like a hostage to the stress of never being able to focus on a single idea.

The mind's lack of focus can feel stressful. It can also be isolating. One of my patients reminded me, "The loneliest place to be is between my ears," because there is no one in your head, just you, in a time machine, jumping from memory to memory, hope to fear and back again.

Many people describe Mindfulness and meditation as pleasant because focusing on the breath going in and out of the body gets them out of the time machine and helps them arrive in the present moment. The present moment can also give them a break from the endless chatter in their head. Connecting to the breath can also connect us to a sense that all things are breathing, all humans, animals, and living things have some aspect of respiration. We are all moving air in and out of our cells. This realization that all beings, not just you, are breathing can decrease the sense of isolation, which was discussed in Chapter 3. Only you know what is happening inside your chatty mind. Returning to your sensory experience is recommended because, unlike thoughts and feelings, your sensory experience is tangible and grounded in the present moment. This is the simple reason that beginning meditation encourages you to focus on the breath.

COUNSELING ACTIVITY – **BECOMING AN OBSERVER**

Remember that cinnamon roll? In this example, you are not going to step into the time machine but stay present and grounded even when the thoughts in your head are complex and hard to sort out. Use your Mindfulness skills of observing your thoughts.

Observe: The smell. Engage your curious mind and ask some questions. Is that a cinnamon roll I smell? Is that something else?

Observe: Your thoughts. I am thinking about my childhood. I am thinking about the past (memory). Isn't that interesting! Was it the smell that triggered this memory?

Observe: The desire to eat a cinnamon roll. Would a cinnamon roll taste good right now? Scan your hunger/fullness level to determine whether eating it would increase your sense of pleasure. Spend some time with the urge to eat a cinnamon roll.

It may be helpful to think of the urge to eat like an ocean wave: It starts slowly. It builds to a peak. Then it passes. A wonderful handout titled "Turning Your Crave into a Wave"[34] by Ronald Thebarge, PhD, is available on The Center for Mindful Eating website.

GOING DEEPER
Debriefing the Observing Thoughts and Emotions Activity

Being able to observe thoughts will help you separate them from your sensory and emotional observations.

1. Take a moment and write down what you liked about the activity.

2. Now list what you would change after trying to observe your thoughts. Create a list, which might help you personally or professionally.

3. Stretch your skills by spending some time in reflection. Ask yourself the following four questions:

- How have I observed this concept being presented? Am I willing to read the handout "Turning Your Crave into a Wave"?

- How can I convey this concept using my words and experiences?

- Have I had an opportunity to teach this concept that cravings have a beginning, middle, and end?

- How will I use the feedback I have received from teaching this concept to advance my counseling practice?

CREATING SPACE FOR YOUR THOUGHTS

Your thoughts are not you. The ability to see yourself separately from your thoughts is one step that can free you from using the Time Machine. As described in the Mindful Eating Map, the first step is nonjudgmentally observing your thought experience as distinct from your sensory experience. It is important to understand that you are not your cravings. You are not your desires, fears, or failures. These are the stories in your head.

The second step is to identify your thought experience as Pleasant, Neutral, or Unpleasant. If being pulled from one thought (say craving) to another thought (maybe fear) is pleasant, that is great to know. If it is neutral, that is good to know, too.

TURN OFF THE MONKEY MIND WHEN EATING

Lots of people would like to learn how to stop their thoughts and cravings and silence the monkey mind. This is just another form of restriction. Instead of telling yourself what you can eat or can't eat, you are now telling yourself what you should crave and shouldn't crave, what you should and shouldn't think and feel. The more you tell yourself **What** You Should Be, **Who** You Should Be, or **How** You Should Be, the more likely shame will follow.[35] Your thoughts create a web of shame that can make the tangle of our behaviors even bigger.

Permission, Freedom, and Space
THE SOLUTION FOR RESTRICTION

There is a lovely Zen riddle that holds the answer to your desire to restrict, limit, and avoid: How do you train an angry bull? Answer: Start with a really big field. Calming your Monkey Mind begins with permission, includes the precious gift of freedom, and, like the bull, needs lots of space.

In the Mindful Eating Map, the first step is to observe what *is* present. This requires permission to notice what *is* present instead of what you *want* to be present. When we pause and notice what is present, many people, myself included, experience things we don't want. I might have wanted hunger to be present instead of the thought of a cinnamon roll. I might have wanted to be calm, instead of frustrated and hooked by a craving that was 20 years old! I might have wanted my observations to be simple, clear, and easy to sort out, instead of a jumble of physical, sensory, and thought information! My desire for my experience to be simple is a craving that is no different from the craving for a cinnamon roll. Mindfulness teaches us how to be present with our thought cravings and our sensory cravings!

The second step is to determine whether your thoughts are Pleasant, Neutral, or Unpleasant. Once you decide, pause and congratulate yourself! You have given yourself permission to tolerate a range of feelings. This permission to have more than one type of thought, one type of feeling, one type of experience is really helpful. This is giving yourself the freedom to have a wide range of thoughts, ideas, and opinions. Once you acknowledge that life comes with lots of thoughts, interests, and ideas, you have opened the door to exploring these thoughts — and maybe even experiencing them!

When you give yourself permission to think a wide range of thoughts, you notice that they take up a lot more room. You need space to process this rich and complex way of thinking. When there is space for thought, your ideas, wants, and desires seem to swirl about. They have a natural buoyancy and these more buoyant thoughts keep coming to the surface. The ones that are more important will rise to the top of the mind.

Deep breath: The bubbling, swirling, churning waters of your mind will calm down if you give it time. Sometimes, an urgency to change can fuel the thought, "What if I forget or miss what is important?" Thoughts such as this can make it harder to observe what is present.

COUNSELING ACTIVITY – EVALUATING THOUGHTS

Explore the two steps of the Mindful Eating Map described above.

DIRECTIONS:
Read this urgent question: "What if I forget or miss what is important?" In the space below, write down some *thoughts* you can observe about this statement. For example, the person is thinking about missing a key piece of information. What are other thoughts that might be related to this?

Thoughts: _____

_____

Next, look at the thoughts you wrote down. Try to determine whether these thoughts are considered Pleasant, Neutral, or Unpleasant.

THOUGHT HABITS AND THERAPY

Many people will seek nutritional counseling as a way to avoid psychotherapy. This avoidance is often unintentional. Honoring your professional limitations and working within your scope of practice is the best way to care for your clients. The "red flag" to guide you is if the clients asks, "**_Why_** am I thinking such unpleasant thoughts?"

"Why" is a therapy question and is beyond this Mindful Eating training. Working with a therapist that is knowledgeable in Mindful Eating may offer the client the necessary support for change. If a client asks you, "**_How_** do I change my thinking about food?" then Mindful Eating is a helpful tool.

GOING DEEPER
Debriefing Evaluating Thoughts Activity

1. Take a moment and write down what you or your client liked about evaluating your thoughts.

2. What didn't you like about the activity? How would you change it to better meet your needs?

3. Stretch your skills by spending some time in reflection. Ask yourself the following three questions:

- How have I observed this concept being presented?
- How can I convey this concept using my own words and experiences?
- How will I use my observations to improve my counseling skills?

COUNSELING ACTIVITY – **THOUGHT COMPASS ON THOUGHT EXPERIENCE**

Consider whether you would like to complete a Thought Compass of this chapter on observing your thought experience. If you do not remember the instructions for Thought Compass, please refer to Chapter 1.

CHAPTER SUMMARY
Thought Experience

HOORAY! Review the counseling tools you just learned.

- Think about observing your thoughts as if you were watching a play, instead of being an actor in the play.
- When listening, describe what the "story" is about.
- When listening, hear the struggle.
- It is OK to "guess" the story and the heart of the struggle. You are providing a complex reflection when you do this.
- One way to create space for your thoughts is to give yourself permission to see them as separate from yourself.

OOPS! Review the struggles you might encounter.

- The problem with observing your thoughts is that, often, you don't even know you are thinking.
- The mind naturally creates "stories" that you can become trapped in.
- The "monkey mind" can be exhausting because it jumps from idea to thought, never allowing you to concentrate.
- Learning to observe your thoughts requires you to tolerate what is present, which is not always pleasant.

TADA! Review the action steps of the chapter.

- Engage in nonjudgmental observation of the current situation.
- Engage in nonjudgmental observation of your thought experience.
- Identify whether your experience is Pleasant, Neutral, or Unpleasant.
- Renew your commitment to daily meditation.
- Renew your commitment to observe your sensory experiences.
- Consider reading *Turning a Crave into a Wave*, handout by Ronald Thebarge, PhD.
- Create a Thought Compass of your own thought experience to help you or create a Thought Compass of what you have learned and discovered so far.

EMPATHIZING - LINDA

"I get so confused when I go shopping with my husband. He will just push the cart and randomly pick up things to eat. These aren't even on the shopping list! And I look at what he has chosen, and I get so frustrated. I want to scream — I mean, COOKIES, ice cream, cake, and chips! I see these things, and my stomach starts turning. I am not even sure if I am hungry, but I know I want to eat them. I know he loves me and wants to support me, but I don't think he has made the connection between the foods we have in the house and my overeating."

— Linda

CHAPTER 6
Emotional Experience

"Mindfulness asks that we don't ignore or pretend angry feelings don't exist. Mindfulness means turning toward them, even when that's difficult."

— CHAR WILKINS, MSW, LCSW, "No Quick Fix," Food for Thought

The last two chapters explored the many things for you to observe. So far, you learned about sensory and thought experience and how they are different. In this chapter, you are going to explore how your emotional experience differs from and overlaps with both sensory and thought experience. As you might have guessed, these three distinct concepts are also closely interwoven, making it harder to separate them into simple concepts.

HOW SENSORY AND EMOTIONAL EXPERIENCES ARE SIMILAR

Have you ever noticed how similar sensory and emotional experiences are? I hadn't until I compared the two.

Hunger: Pangs, growling, grumbling, emptiness, gnawing, queasy feeling, tiredness, low energy, weakness, irritability, mild headache, difficulty concentrating, thinking, or making decisions.

Sadness: Stomach sensation or ***pangs, grumbling, emptiness, gnawing, queasy feeling, tiredness, low energy, irritability***, emotionally frailty, ***difficulty concentrating, thinking, or making decisions.***

What did you notice when you compared the list? It is a bit shocking how similar they are. If you are not used to observing your emotional experience, you might think you are hungry when actually you are sad, or you might think you are sad when actually you are hungry. As you notice how closely intertwined your sensory, thought, and emotions are, it is easy to empathize with how you and others can get confused.

If you are unaware that your emotions generate a physical experience, it gets even more confusing. The best way to observe this is to try the following activity.

COUNSELING ACTIVITY – WHERE YOUR EMOTIONS ARE FELT

DIRECTIONS: Take five deep breaths. Try to do this activity when you are physically comfortable. Read the list of emotions in Table 3. After each emotion, see if you can identify the place in/on the body where you might feel it. Many people find it helpful to touch the body part. Write down the area you touched. The first two feelings are provided as an example.

Feeling	Where is it felt in your body?	Feeling	Where is it felt in your body?
Afraid	Chest	*Affectionate*	Heart Area
Annoyed		*Engaged*	
Angry		*Hopeful*	
Aversion		*Confident*	
Confused		*Excited*	
Disconnected		*Grateful*	
Disquieted		*Inspired*	
Embarrassed		*Joyful*	
Fatigued		*Exhilarated*	
Pain		*Peaceful*	
Sad		*Refreshed*	
Tense			
Vulnerable			
Yearning			

The overlap between your sensory and emotional experience can create confusion or misunderstanding, which can generate a feeling of uncertainty. For many people, feeling confused or uncertain is not a pleasant experience. Learning to identify unpleasant experiences is part of Mindful Eating.

Individuals who eat mindfully are able to recognize a feeling as unpleasant without adding any story, opinion, or value to the experience. Recognizing unpleasant feelings provides you a choice: to keep eating something that wasn't great, or to modify the choice to increase your enjoyment.

In Mindful Eating, identifying whether an experience is Pleasant, Neutral, or Unpleasant is one step in a two-step process. The second step is developing the ability to stop or to change the eating experience when it no longer suits you. This means that the person who eats mindfully not only has the *intention* to stop eating when it is unpleasant, but also *acts* on this information! This is summarized in Steps 4a and 4b of the Mindful Eating Map.

NOT ALL EXPERIENCES ARE PLEASANT

Life is not always pleasant, and eating experiences will not all be pleasant. This is because not all feelings are pleasant. To help you explain this concept, imagine a box of crayons with 64 colors. Some colors you love, some you dislike, and there are some that you don't even think about — for example, tan and black. Feelings are a lot like this box of crayons. Some feelings are hard to be present with because you don't like them. Some are easy because you enjoy them, and there are some you don't think about. Having the ability to tolerate different feelings means you can choose any color in that box of 64 crayons. If you can tolerate only one type of feeling, say only the "green" feelings, then you now can't tolerate the experience of reds, yellows, blues, purples, grays, tans, or any of those funny-named colors like Twilight Tangerine. The ability to tolerate a wide spectrum of feelings makes life colorful, rich, complex, and interesting. The same is true with eating. The ability to experience the feelings of eating a variety of foods, tastes, and flavors makes eating interesting, rich, complex, and nutritious!

TOLERATING VS. ENJOYING

Like life, Mindful Eating won't make food a magical experience filled with rainbows and butterflies. Sometimes, our food choices fall somewhere between amazing and terrible. The middle ground can feel pretty dull. Why would anyone want you to tolerate a food choice? Because what you enjoy is subjective and can change moment to moment. One day, a meal is fine (not great, but OK), and the next day, it is delicious! A week later, the same delicious meal isn't enjoyable at all! Thinking that all meals "should" taste amazing is unrealistic — not only unrealistic, but it can also lead to the same judgmental behavior associated with guilt, blame, and shame.

Still, just because a meal doesn't taste AMAZING doesn't mean the eating experience is not enjoyable. Your sensory experience, the actual taste of the food, is only one part of your overall experience. You can now observe your thoughts and feelings, and (this is the exciting part) determine whether they are adding enjoyment to the meal or taking enjoyment away. Most people don't want to overanalyze each aspect of a meal, so it is easier to think of your experience as Pleasant, Neutral, or Unpleasant.

COUNSELING ACTIVITY – **EVALUATING YOUR FEELINGS**

0   1   2   3   4   5   6   7   8   9   10

unpleasant   **neutral**   **pleasant**

Image 6

Image 6 is a scale from 0 (Unpleasant) to 10 (Pleasant). Use this to rate your feelings at your next meal or snack.

DIRECTIONS: Rate your feelings *before* your next meal or snack. Ask those open-ended questions: How did I feel before I started to eat? n what way are my feelings before the meal adding an undesired flavor to my meal or snack?

Take two bites, and re-evaluate your feelings. Ask yourself, "Is there anything I can do, right now, to help this eating experience be more pleasant?" Check in with your feelings.

GOING DEEPER
Debriefing Evaluating Your Feelings Activity

1. Take a moment and write down what was beneficial about evaluating your feelings before a meal or snack.

2. What didn't you like about the activity? How would you change it to better meet your needs?

3. Stretch your skills by spending some time in reflection. Ask yourself the following four questions:

- How have I heard this concept being presented?
- How can I convey this concept using my own words and experiences?
- Have I had an opportunity to observe this concept? Do I want to teach this concept at a session, class, or group?
- After I teach this, how will I use my observations to improve my counseling skills?

THE FUNNY THING ABOUT FEELINGS

Some feelings are more tolerable than others. There are loads of reasons you can tolerate a feeling better than your friend, partner, or neighbor can. Regardless of your natural ability, you can increase your tolerance of feelings by engaging in the mindfulness practice of observation. It is harder to watch your feelings than it is to watch your thoughts or physical sensations because you feel your feelings. Making the connection between your feelings and a physical response can change how you respond to this information.

For example, if you are feeling afraid, and this is making it hard to breathe, your physical response to the feeling of fear makes it harder, if not impossible, to tolerate. Not being able to breathe is a frightening experience, and it makes total sense to advocate for yourself immediately! A less-extreme example may better convey where mindful observation can be helpful. For example, you do a quick check-in and notice that you are a 3 on the feelings-evaluation scale. Refer to Image 6 to assist you in your evaluation. You observe that you are feeling uncertain. Your stomach is a bit cramped, and your shoulders are raised toward your ears. You decide to pause and take five deep breaths, filling your belly with air and your mind with the intention to lower your shoulders. Now recheck your experience. If the experience has decreased in enjoyment and dropped from a 3 to a 2 or 1, then the situation is clearly unpleasant. If the experience still rates as a 3, then you may decide whether there is a change possible, for example, taking a break or shifting your sitting position. If you rated the experience as 4 or above, then you just discovered a tool that can help you make a feeling on the verge of being unpleasant become a neutral experience.

COUNSELING ACTIVITY – **FEELING YOUR FEELINGS**

Here is what Linda said about feeling her feelings.

I have seen dietitians in the past who are trying to get me to connect with my feelings and see the connection. In all honesty, I got confused. I was too embarrassed to explain that I got confused, especially because so many people were talking about how powerful the experience was. You are the first person I have told about this. I think you knowing this will help us make progress. I eat when I am upset, and I don't understand how to separate my feelings from my eating! I can never tell if this headache is hunger, low blood sugar, or actually a headache. If I don't figure this out, I will never get better. I know that my blood sugar is high after I "eat my heart out."

Review the options to try to help Linda with either Step 1 or Step 2 of the Mindful Eating Map.

Step 1
Stretch your ability to engage in nonjudgmental observation of the three areas of the current situation.

- **a.** Sensory experience: Taste, sight, sound, feel, hunger, fullness, satiety, wellness, illness, pain, discomfort, etc.
- **b.** Thought experience.
- **c.** Emotional experience.

Step 2
Try to categorize your observations as Pleasant, Neutral/Unsure, or Unpleasant.

DIRECTIONS: Complete the following questions using the Mindful Eating Map.

Stretch your ability to engage in nonjudgmental observation of the current situation.

- _____
- _____
- _____

What are the sensory experiences described by Linda? Taste, sight, sound, feel, hunger, fullness, satiety, wellness, illness, pain, discomfort etc.

- _____
- _____
- _____

What are the thought experiences described by Linda?

- _____
- _____
- _____

What are the emotional experiences described by Linda?

- _____
- _____
- _____

How would you categorize Linda's overall experience with noticing her feelings?

Pleasant, Neutral/Unsure, or Unpleasant. Use your answer to write down some counseling questions that clarify her desire to change.

- _____
- _____
- _____

DIRECTIONS: Write a few reflections using Linda's dialog.

Simple reflection helps the client know that you are listening.

- _____
- _____
- _____

Complex reflection helps the client know you understand the larger issue, which in this chapter is how to process all of the available emotional information.

- _____
- _____
- _____

Summarize the main point or focus of the dialog you would like to have with Linda.

- _____
- _____
- _____

GOING DEEPER
Debriefing the Feeling Your Feelings Activity

1. Take a moment and write down what you liked about the *Feeling Your Feelings* Activity.

2. What questions arose about the activity? How would you change it to better meet your needs?

3. Stretch your skills by spending some time in reflection. Ask yourself the following four questions:

- Have you made the connection between emotions and sensory experience?
- Where can I learn more about this concept?
- Do I wish to convey this concept using my own words and experiences?
- How will this activity improve my counseling skills?

PERMISSION IS SURPRISINGLY POWERFUL

Giving yourself permission to observe how you feel your feelings also gives you permission to have more than one feeling at the same time. Once you acknowledge that life comes with lots of feelings, you open the door to something unexpected: emotional freedom. You are no longer required to feel a specific way about food. You are free to like a food one day and dislike it the next. You are allowed to be OK with a choice one moment and to change your mind the next!

Remember when I compared feelings to colors? When you give yourself permission to choose any color, you don't have to choose your favorite color or a color that someone else likes. You have permission to choose any color. Colors aren't right or wrong. If someone said that you were "wrong" for liking a specific color, what would you do? You might think, "You're joking, right?" What if you used the same logic with food? What if there weren't "good" or "bad" food choices? What if food was more like those crayon colors, and you could make a choice because it felt good to you? Would that change your food and eating choices?

Many clients don't realize how their feelings affect their food and eating choices. Feelings like fear, doubt, aversion, confidence, excitement, and peacefulness register in the body. Emotional experiences can be confused with physical, or sensory, experiences. Learning how to observe your feelings is helpful, but it is different from thinking about them or even trying to outthink them. Observing means watching your feelings come and go, like the clouds in the sky or the waves of the ocean.

Feelings can also influence, in obvious and subtle ways, what foods are available in the home and which are selected during a meal. Learning to observe your feelings can help you make connections between what you are feeling and what you choose to eat.

THE SPACE FOR YOUR FEELINGS

In Chapter 4, you learned to notice whether a food was Beckoning or Humming. I learned a useful trick from Jean Fain, LICSW, during her self-compassion workshop. In the workshop, she instructed participants to "Place your hand over your heart and ask, Is my heart humming for something?" In my own retreat, I suggest placing your cupped hands in front of you as if you were asking someone to place a gift in them. If you are humming, you are ready to receive the gift of this food. Check in with your deeper wisdom, and listen for whether this food is just what your body needs at this moment. If it isn't just what your body needs at this moment, what is your body asking for? What would hum inside of you? What would feel like a welcome gift?

The willingness to make the 13-inch journey from your head to your heart and actually feel your feelings begins the next Mindful Eating phase — listening to the compassionate wisdom inside you. Try to imagine this wisdom as the trust you feel when you listen and are truly mindful. The information that arises allows you to honor your direct experience, to be genuine and authentic to the wide range of emotions that are present.

When you give yourself permission to feel a range of emotions, you notice that they take up a lot more room. You need space to process this rich and complex experience. When there is space, your feelings, ideas, wants, and desires seem to swirl about. Pause and notice that your feelings seem to have a natural buoyancy to them, that they keep coming back! The ability to sit back and observe allows you notice the ones that are more important, because they rise to the top of the mind.

The intention of Mindfulness is to help you "welcome" your feelings and increase your acceptance of them. "The Guest House," written by Sufi poet Rumi, explains this beautifully. It is often used as a teaching tool in Mindfulness-based stress reduction (MBSR).

The Guest House

This being human is a guest house.
Every morning a new arrival.

A joy, a depression, a meanness,
some momentary awareness comes
as an unexpected visitor.

Welcome and entertain them all!
Even if they are a crowd of sorrows,
who violently sweep your house
empty of its furniture,
still, treat each guest honorably.

He may be clearing you out
for some new delight.

The dark thought, the shame, the malice.
Meet them at the door laughing
and invite them in.

Be grateful for whatever comes.
Because each has been sent
as a guide from beyond.

— Jellaludin Rumi (translation by Coleman Barks)

This poem describes an opportunity for reflection. Some feelings are powerful forces "who violently sweep your house empty of its furniture." Chances are you have already had your house emptied by those powerful emotions!

Emotional upheaval can be so painful that you think, "I don't want to experience this ever again!" This is another place where Mindfulness can help. Ask yourself, "Do I think my feelings or do I feel my feelings?" As hard as you might try to think about them, you have to feel your feelings. In Chapter 3, I talked about making the 13-inch journey, from your head to your heart. It takes courage to keep your heart open, to be vulnerable. In her TED talk *Listening to Shame*, Brené Brown describes how vulnerability is necessary to living a whole-hearted life! This means that the 13-inch journey is both essential AND hard.

CREATING CONDITIONS FOR ACCEPTANCE

Letting go of emotionally triggering experiences is not easy, but your ability to do this will increase with practice. What do you do while you practice? Create conditions where you are **more likely** to be successful. Mindful Eating stresses that awareness of a situation can help you create the conditions for a change to occur. Mindful Eating training is not about creating a to-do list, such as eat in silence, chew your food 20 times, eat slowly, eat only with chop sticks, etc. Mindful Eating asks that you determine what conditions need to be present for you to be aware of the enjoyment you are getting from your meal or snack. Can you be aware if you are eating quickly? If yes, terrific. If no, it makes it harder for you to taste and enjoy your meal, this is great to know. This is a critical point to understand, and it is worth repeating:

Focus on conditions necessary for awareness of enjoyment to arise.

What are the conditions necessary for awareness of enjoyment to arise for you? Brian Wansink, PhD, author of *Mindless Eating*, discusses the many environments that contribute to mindless eating. Triggers can be plate size, food is left out, other people are eating. MindlessEating.org offers ways to remove mindless-eating cues and triggers. Wansink's book not only makes clear the connections between the environmental cues and unconscious behavioral habits that can promote mindless, reactive eating, but also is very funny!

Is eating less mindlessly the same as eating mindfully? No, Mindful Eating trains the mind to become aware of sensory, cognitive, and emotional experiences — very different from environmental changes such as eating on a smaller plate and tucking snacks out of sight.

Mindfulness looks at more than your physical environment. It explores your internal environment – the rich sensory experience, thoughts, and feelings — and asks, What conditions are necessary for you to observe these? What are the patterns you observe? What tiny choice can you make to enjoy your experience a little bit more? The decision to recognize and choose enjoyment is not tied to an outcome like size, weight loss, or calories.

Creating the conditions for you to notice your feelings is often about creating space apart from the rush and bustle of life. In Chapter 4, you were introduced to the graphic *The Tree of Contemplative Practices*. Here is a way to understand and use the tree graphic.

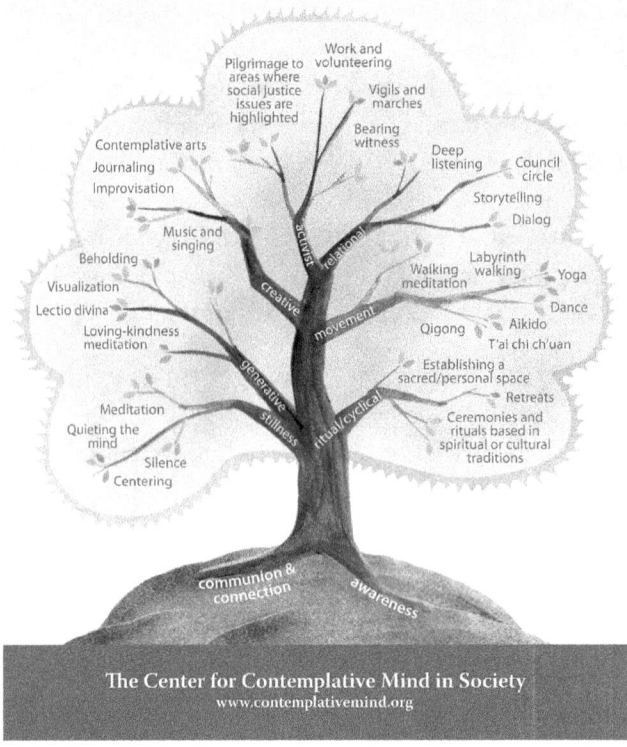

The roots symbolize the two foundations of all contemplative practices:

- The first is communion and connection.
- The second is awareness.

The branches represent different groupings of practices:

- Stillness — Meditation can quiet the mind and body and develop calmness and focus.
- Generative — Different forms share the common intent of generating thoughts and feelings, such as devotion and compassion.
- Creative — Thoughts and feelings can be expressed through music, journaling, and art.
- Activist – Practice includes bearing witness, vigils, volunteering, and pilgrimages.
- Relational — Deep listening, storytelling, council circles, etc.
- Movement — Tai chi, yoga, Qigong, walking meditation.
- Ritual/cyclical — Retreats and rituals.

Activities such as gardening or eating may be understood to be contemplative practices when done with the intent of cultivating awareness and wisdom.

If you visit the website http://www.contemplativemind.org/practices/tree, you can download a free blank tree that you can customize to include your practices.

Engaging in contemplative practices on a regular and consistent basis creates the conditions for awareness of your emotional triggers to arise. By practicing these behaviors, you give yourself many more chances for wisdom and understanding to arise.

COUNSELING ACTIVITY – USING THE MINDFUL EATING MAP

DIRECTIONS: Read Linda's statement below. Then reflect on how Mindful Eating might assist her. Refer back to Chapter 3 to use EARS or DARN to identify the change talk that will help the client move out of her repetitive behavioral cycle.

Oh my gosh, I can always tell what I was feeling when I went shopping. If there were salad and loads of fresh vegetables, chances are I felt guilty and was shopping after a binge. You know, "You can't have anything but the most healthiest foods because look at all that you just ate!"

If there are bread, crackers, or cookies in the house, I have either been really "good" so I can "have a little," or I have just quit the diet, and I am thinking, "Who cares? You blew it, Linda. Get a French bread baguette, too!"

Review of the options to help Linda with Step 1 or Step 2 of the Mindful Eating Map.

Step 1
Stretch your ability to engage in nonjudgmental observation of the current situation, in three areas of focus:

- **a.** Sensory experience: taste, sight, sound, feel, hunger, fullness, satiety, wellness, illness, pain, discomfort, etc.
- **b.** Thought experience.
- **c.** Emotional experience.

Step 2
Categorize your observations as Pleasant, Neutral/Unsure, or Unpleasant.

DIRECTIONS: Complete the following questions using the Mindful Eating Map.

Describe nonjudgmentally Linda's observation of the current situation.

- _____
- _____
- _____

Are there any sensory experiences? Taste, sight, sound, feel, hunger, fullness, satiety, wellness, illness, pain, discomfort, etc.

- _____
- _____
- _____

What are the thought experiences described by Linda?

- _____
- _____
- _____

What are the emotional experiences described by Linda?

- _____
- _____
- _____

How would you categorize Linda's overall experience with her feelings? Pleasant, Neutral/Unsure, or Unpleasant. Use your answer to write down some counseling questions that clarify her desire to change.

- _____
- _____
- _____

DIRECTIONS: Complete the following reflection using Linda's dialog.

Write a few simple reflections to help the Linda know that you are listening.

- _____
- _____
- _____

Write a few complex reflections to help Linda know you understand her larger issue.

- _____
- _____
- _____

Summarize the main point or focus of Linda's statement.

- _____
- _____
- _____

GOING DEEPER
Debriefing Using the Mindful Eating Map Activity

1. Take a moment and write down what you or your client liked about using the Mindful Eating Map.

2. What was lacking about the activity? How would you change it to better meet your needs?

3. Stretch your skills by spending some time in reflection. Ask yourself the following four questions:

- How have I observed this concept of feeling my feelings presented?
- How can I convey this concept using my own words and experiences?
- Where can I observe this concept being presented?
- Will using this concept improve my counseling skills?

HOW YOUR GUT GETS IN THE WAY

Many of our choices are not based on knowledge, but on more subtle information.

Your "gut" response to a situation is either to go toward a choice or to move away from a choice. For example, if I offered you some kale chips, would you move toward them? If the thought of kale chips makes you say, "Yum," and you feel your salivary glands activate, you are likely to move toward that choice. However, if these dark green crisps aren't familiar or aren't on your list of delicious foods, you might say, "No, thank you," and move away from this choice. The desire to move toward or away from a choice is so automatic that it may be unconscious.

Neuroscientist Daniel Siegel, MD, offers the analogy of a car to understand how a person unconsciously enters into a choice situation. If a person is moving toward something, it is like giving the car some gas. If you're pressing the gas pedal, you are moving toward a choice. If you don't wish to move toward something, you use the brake. The gas and brake analogy is helpful for seeing this unconscious force behind the choice. You can modify this analogy for a patient with a simple kinesthetic-learning technique using your hands.

COUNSELING ACTIVITY – **GAS, BRAKE, OR BOTH?**

Look at a choice, such as eating kale chips. Now place your hands in the stop position. Ask yourself if the stop gesture is how you feel about eating the kale chips. Now try turning your hands over, palms up, in the receiving position. Ask yourself if this accepting position is how you feel about the kale chips. Now turn one hand to the stop position and the other hand to the accepting position, and ask yourself if this mix of emotions is what you feel about kale chips.

How a person responds to a situation is often a mix of emotions. It isn't as simple as go or stop, gas or brake. Emotions are mixed, and you may find you have the brake and gas on at the same time. This creates the feeling of being stuck.

GOING DEEPER
Debriefing Feeling Stuck

Take a moment and list what was helpful from doing this activity. Did it help to use your hands and imagine how you would respond to kale chips? Was it helpful to realize that you can experience both a desire to come toward and to move away from a food, creating a sense of feeling stuck?

1. Take a moment to write down what you liked about the activity.

2. Now list what you would change. Remain nonjudgmental regarding the response. All awareness is helpful, even if you found no benefit from the activity.

3. Stretch your skills by spending some time in reflection. Ask yourself the following three questions:

- How have I observed being stuck?
- How can I convey being stuck using my own words and experiences?
- How can I use my observations to improve my counseling skills?

COUNSELING ACTIVITY – **THOUGHT COMPASS EMOTIONS**

Consider whether you would like to complete a Thought Compass of this chapter about observing your feelings. (Brief review for making a Thought Compass: Draw four lines from the center concept, Mindful Eating and Feelings, that you write inside the circle. Now, think back on the chapter and write four subtopics. Continue to expand your Thought Compass until you have exhausted your ideas.) Take a moment to see connections, patterns, or overlapping ideas.

CHAPTER SUMMARY
Emotional Experience

HOORAY! Review the counseling tools you just learned.

- Connecting your feelings to a part of the body.
- Tolerating your feelings begins with cultivating curiosity and compassion for all feelings.
- Using Steps 1 and 2 of the Mindful Eating Map.
- Reviewing contemplative practices.
- The Gas and Brake activity, which can help a client notice his "gut" reaction to a situation.

OOPS! Review the struggles you might encounter.

- There is often overlap among sensory information, cognitive information, and emotional information.
- This overlap can make it challenging to distinguish between emotional experiences, like being upset, and physical hunger.
- Not all emotions are pleasant, which requires you to evaluate the feelings you can tolerate and identify ways to move toward acceptance.
- It is easy to judge unpleasant feelings as "bad" or "wrong" when, in fact, feelings are simply present.
- It is tempting to place unpleasant feelings in a box, instead of giving yourself permission to feel your feelings and to have the necessary space to accept them.
- Focusing on situations and tips to control your feelings is not the goal of Mindful Eating.

TADA! Review the action steps of the chapter.

- Engage in nonjudgmental observation of the current situation.
- Identify whether the current situation is Pleasant, Neutral, or Unpleasant.
- Engage in nonjudgmental observation of sensory experience: taste, sight, sound, feel, hunger, fullness, satiety, etc.
- Identify whether a sensory experience is Pleasant, Neutral, or Unpleasant.
- Engage in nonjudgmental observation of thought experience.
- Identify whether your thought experience is Pleasant, Neutral, or Unpleasant.
- Complete the Contemplative Tree activity.
- Create a Thought Compass of this chapter.

SECTION THREE

Identifying Your Needs, Creating Your Intention, Advocating for Your Practice, Teaching Your Passion

INTRODUCTION TO
Section Three

In Section Three, you will spend some time identifying your needs. Once you know what you need, you can create your intention to meet this need. You learned in Chapter 3 that creating a clear intention is very powerful. It is true, you won't learn to walk on water, but you now know that even if your actions are imperfect, having an intention that is grounded in kindness and care changes a person in amazing ways. Section Three will provide support and ideas for you to teach Mindful Eating in a more effective way.

HOW THIS SECTION IS SET UP

In Chapter 7, you will learn more about identifying your nutritional, health, and wellness needs with self-compassion. Lessons from Chapter 6 regarding feelings will be applied to help you identify your personals needs. In Step 3 of the Mindful Eating Map, you will notice additional concepts that can help you focus on self-compassion for yourself and others.

In Chapter 8, you will explore how to set your intention to reduce the negative experience associated with your unmet needs by reviewing three common problems, called "poisons."

Chapter 9 will help you create a personalized Mindful Eating practice. Here you will learn about a powerful tool called The Practice Planning Worksheet, which will move you from intentions to clear and actionable goals. The Practice Planning Worksheet, or PPW, can help you learn how to engage in Step 5 of the Mindful Eating Map, ***Advocate for yourself*** and all living beings ***ethically***.

Chapter 10 offers a Motivational Interviewing model for teaching Mindful Eating that makes groups and classes exciting, fun, and effective! In this chapter, you will have a chance to review the many concepts presented and to choose the ideas that resonate deeply with you.

EMPATHIZING - JEROME

"My mother doesn't know what to do with me. She is angry at me about my pickiness, and it frustrates her. I know that I make her crazy. I am not like my sister, who will eat anything. My mother jokes, 'At least I have one easy child,' and I know she isn't talking about me. I really should eat more and not be so fussy at dinner, like my sister. I think people want me to be "brave" and 'act older' when it comes to eating."

— Jerome

CHAPTER 7

Identifying Your Needs

"Habits are patterns of behavior that we learn to do with little attention. It is a wonder and gift that our brains are capable of developing habits. However, when we rely on them too much, habits rob us of choice."

— Molly Kellogg, RD, LCSW, "Choosing Your Way to Mindfulness," Food for Thought

So far in your journey using the Mindful Eating Map, you have had a chance to discover, explore, and even play with some new skills. In Step 1, you stretched your ability to engage in nonjudgmental observation of the current situation. Now you can nonjudgmentally observe either sensory, thought, or emotional experience. This distinction will help you in this chapter, which explores your needs.

In Step 2, you determined whether your experience was Pleasant, Neutral/Unsure, or Unpleasant. Your ability to identify your current experience provides the motivation necessary to take action.

It is time to explore Step 3, which asks you to "identify your personal needs with self-compassion." Step 3 has two parts: Personal Needs, and Needs and Feelings.

MINDFUL EATING MAP STEP 3, PART ONE: *Personal Needs*

Your mind may tell you there is someone somewhere who doesn't need a thing, but that is just a story, often fueled by shame. If it is hard to verbalize your needs, reach into your bag of self-compassion and fish out the common-humanity aspect of Step 3. All humans have needs – not just you.

Your needs are real, and they deserve your time, attention, and effort. They also change throughout your life, and thus, understanding your needs can seem elusive. Your needs are physical, emotional, and mental. In this chapter, we will use two models to look at your needs. The first is "The Healthy Mind Platter" Dan Siegel, MD,. The second is the "Nonviolent Communication" method created by Marshall Rosenberg, PhD, of the Center for Nonviolent Communication. The NVC model will help you not only meet your needs, but also verbalize your needs to other people.

MENTAL WELLNESS

People often forget each part of the body that has its own set of requirements. One part of the body that is important to consider is the brain. Your brain (the physical organ) is where your mind (the chemical connections) operates your body. Siegel, a neuroscientist and one of my professional heroes, writes about mental wellness[39] and the advantages of keeping the brain healthy. To do this, he identifies seven areas of importance: Sleep Time, Physical Time, Focus Time, Time-in, Downtime, Play Time, Connecting Time.

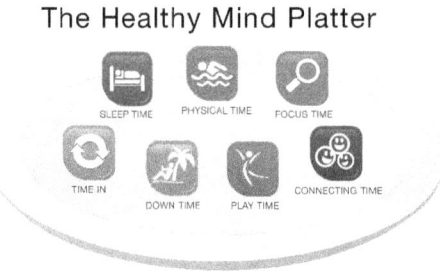

The Healthy Mind Platter, for Optimal Brain Matter

To optimize brain matter and create well-being, Siegel encourages daily engagement in the seven essential mental activities. Those that overlap with the practice of Mindful Eating are underlined.

Sleep Time: When you give the brain the rest it needs, your consolidate learning and recover from the experiences of the day.

Physical Time: When you move your body — aerobically, if medically possible — you strengthen the brain in measurable ways.

Focus Time: When you focus on tasks in a goal-oriented way, you take on challenges that make deep connections in the brain. Putting aside distractions and giving yourself permission to focus is a way to nourish your brain — and also is part of Mindful Eating.

Time In: When you engage in contemplative practices — quietly reflecting internally, focusing on sensations, images, feelings, and thoughts — you help the brain to better integrate. In Mindful Eating, two examples of nourishing your brain are meditation and savoring the bite.

Downtime: When you give yourself a chance to day-dream, to be without any specific goal, to let your mind wander and relax, you are helping the brain recharge.

Play Time: When you allow yourselves to laugh, be spontaneous, be creative, to enjoy novel experiences, you help make new connections in the brain. By now, you can guess that having fun in the kitchen is a great way to express creativity, try new things, and have some fun!

Connecting Time: Connecting with other people, ideally in person, and taking time to appreciate your connection to the natural world around you helps you activate and reinforce the brain's relational circuitry. Mealtimes are a natural way to connect with the people in your life!

As you can see, five of the seven activities for a healthy brain can be achieved with Mindful Eating! This overlap is exciting because it is showing that the more mindful you are with food and eating, the healthier your brain becomes!

COUNSELING ACTIVITY – **HEALTHY MIND PLATTER**

DIRECTIONS: Below are the seven essentials of a healthy mind. Take a moment, and rate how you feel you are meeting these needs — from 1 (poorly) to 10 (well). After each evaluation, ask yourself, "What options are present?" to either continue your current effort, or increase or decrease it. Include activities, behaviors, and choices to keep your brain healthy and help your mind think and function optimally.

Sleep Time:
What options are present?

Physical Time:
What options are present?

Focus Time:
What options are present?

Time In:
What options are present?

Downtime:
What options are present?

Play Time:
What options are present?

Connecting Time:
What options are present?

GOING DEEPER
Debriefing the Healthy Mind Platter Activity

1. Take a moment and write down what you liked about using the Healthy Mind Platter.

2. What didn't you like about the activity? How would you change it to better meet your needs? Do you want to change your counseling to consider the needs of your brain?

3. Stretch your skills by spending some time in reflection. Ask yourself the following four questions:

- Have I thought about what my brain needs to be healthy?

- Are there other neuroscientists that I would like to consider reading? Examples include Rick Hanson, Sandra Aamodt, Rebecca Gladding, or Judson Brewer.

- How can I convey this concept using my own words and experiences?

- How will I use the feedback I have received from observation to improve my counseling skills?

STEP 3, PART TWO: Needs and Feelings

FEELINGS AS A GATEWAY TO YOUR NEEDS

Your feelings can be a guide to understanding your needs. In the following activity, explore how your feelings are different when your needs are satisfied and when they are not satisfied. The process comes from The Center for Nonviolent Communication,[40] www.CNVC.org, and can help you discover, explore, and challenge your needs and determine whether they are being met or unmet in a mindful way.

COUNSELING ACTIVITY – INTRODUCTION TO NONVIOLENT COMMUNICATION

Below is A List of Feelings that arise when your needs are satisfied.[41] Take a moment and highlight the feelings that are present — or as Rosenberg, creator of Nonviolent Communication, describes it, "What's alive in you?"

AFFECTIONATE	ENGAGED	PEACEFUL	EXHILARATED	EXCITED
compassionate	absorbed	calm	blissful	amazed
friendly	alert	clear-headed	ecstatic	animated
loving	curious	comfortable	elated	ardent
open-hearted	engrossed	centered	enthralled	aroused
sympathetic	enchanted	content	exuberant	astonished
tender	entranced	equanimous	radiant	dazzled
warm	fascinated	fulfilled	rapturous	eager
HOPEFUL	interested	mellow	thrilled	energetic
expectant	intrigued	quiet	**EXHILARATED**	enthusiastic
encouraged	involved	relaxed	blissful	giddy
optimistic	spellbound	relieved	ecstatic	invigorated
CONFIDENT	stimulated	satisfied	elated	lively
empowered	**GRATEFUL**	serene	enthralled	passionate
open	appreciative	still	exuberant	surprised
proud	moved	tranquil	radiant	vibrant
safe	thankful	tickled	rapturous	**REFRESHED**
secure	touched	**JOYFUL**	thrilled	enlivened
	INSPIRED	amused		rejuvenated
	amazed	delighted		renewed
	awed	glad		rested
	wonder	happy		restored
		jubilant		revived
		pleased		

Below is another list of feelings, but these are likely present when your needs are not satisfied. Use a highlighter to identify those emotions that are present in you.

AFRAID	**ANNOYED**	**ANGRY**	**CONFUSED**	**DISCONNECTED**
apprehensive	aggravated	enraged	ambivalent	alienated
dread	dismayed	furious	baffled	aloof
foreboding	disgruntled	incensed	bewildered	apathetic
frightened	displeased	indignant	dazed	bored
mistrustful	exasperated	irate	hesitant	cold
panicked	frustrated	livid	lost	detached
petrified	impatient	outraged	mystified	distant
scared	irritated	resentful	perplexed	distracted
suspicious	irked	**AVERSION**	puzzled	indifferent
terrified	**EMBARRASSED**	animosity	torn	numb
wary	ashamed	appalled	**PAIN**	removed
worried	chagrined	contempt	agony	uninterested
SAD	flustered	disgusted	anguished	withdrawn
depressed	guilty	dislike	bereaved	**DISQUIET**
dejected	mortified	hate	devastated	agitated
despair	self-conscious	horrified	grief	alarmed
despondent	**FATIGUE**	hostile	heartbroken	discombobulated
disappointed	beat	repulsed	hurt	disconcerted
discouraged	burnt out	**TENSE**	lonely	disturbed
disheartened	depleted	anxious	miserable	perturbed
forlorn	exhausted	cranky	regretful	rattled
gloomy	lethargic	distressed	remorseful	restless
heavy hearted	listless	distraught	**VULNERABLE**	shocked
hopeless	sleepy	edgy	fragile	startled
melancholy	tired	fidgety	guarded	surprised
unhappy	weary	frazzled	helpless	troubled
wretched	worn out	irritable	insecure	turbulent
YEARNING		jittery	leery	turmoil
envious		nervous	reserved	uncomfortable
jealous		overwhelmed	sensitive	uneasy
longing		restless	shaky	unnerved
nostalgic		stressed out		unsettled
pining				upset
wistful				

Now consider: What are the behaviors or situations that helped you feel satisfied? What are the behaviors or situations that seemed to promote less-satisfied feelings?

Review both of these lists and ask:

- Could these feelings be the result of you meeting your needs? What are you doing that is working? Do you want to keep doing this behavior? If you do want to keep going, really connect with the benefits that you are experiencing.

- Could these feelings be the result of you NOT meeting your needs. What are you doing that could be shifted, adapted or changed to better meet your needs?

Observing your feelings will help you begin to notice patterns, which can lead you to behaviors that are renewing and helpful, or can alert you to behaviors that are draining and harmful. You will notice a pattern as you commit to observing or becoming mindful of situations.

GOING DEEPER
Debriefing the List of Feelings Activity

1. Take a moment and write down what you liked about using the List of Feelings.
2. What didn't you like about the activity? How would you change it to better meet your needs?
3. Stretch your skills by spending some time in reflection. Ask yourself the following four questions:

- How have I observed this concept being presented?
- Do I wish to learn more about my needs?
- How would I go about that? What process or resources would assist me?
- Does this activity deepen my counseling skills

NEEDS, FEELINGS, AND COUNSELING

You are aware that each person on this planet has needs. These needs can be explained in a number of ways. One way is to look at a person's physical needs, which include the behaviors and situations for a healthy mind. Another way is to look at a person's feelings, recognizing that the feelings that arise when your needs are satisfied seem to be more pleasant than the feelings that arise when your needs are not satisfied. Your needs act like an emotional compass, helping you become mindful that your needs are or are not being met. Both of these tools can be used to help you discover the larger need when working with clients.

Hold in your mind the truth that it is so much easier to *tell* yourself what you need than it is to ask yourself what you need. Many people think they need things to be easier, so they seek out mental shortcuts and crave simple answers. Unfortunately, telling yourself what you need is not a shortcut to mental health, a better life, or Mindfulness. Without adequate reflection, the habit of telling yourself what you need will cause you to become stuck in a habitual pattern of thinking. Craving the simple answer is just another kind of craving. It is hard to accept that life is complex and challenging and that no one knows what you need except you. This is why establishing a consistent time for reflection, via meditation, journaling, and yoga, is important. These periods of reflection will help you see your life as it is, including the complexities and challenges. It will help you separate your needs from these hard-to-see habitual cravings. It will help you stop reacting to the overt and subtle stories that inhabit your head. Reflection keeps the big picture in mind, while you focus on the smaller, day-to-day tasks that can be overwhelming. While this is true for someone with positive mental health, if one is depressed, this is even tougher to see. The help of a trained counselor is key!

When working with clients, the ability to engage in complex reflection is important. Complex reflections help the client know you understand them, their problems, their issues. In the next activity, you will use complex reflections to help Jerome explore and identify his deeper needs.

COUNSELING ACTIVITY – EXPLORING FEELINGS USING COMPLEX REFLECTIONS

Jerome offered this comment:

I started to think about what you said, you know, about the pain in my stomach. People would tell me, "You must be hungry," but my stomach hurt so much, I never felt hungry. When you asked me, "Could the pain be hunger?"

I knew it wasn't. I was so annoyed at you. In the office you asked me, "What are your ideas to make the pain less?" And I didn't know. I am confused and upset that I have to come here. I ate those crackers because I didn't know what else to do. But those crackers seemed to help, and that surprised me.

DIRECTIONS: Using Jerome's comment, write down the feelings that he might be experiencing. You can refer to the list of feelings above. Remember, these could be feelings from his needs being met or unmet.

_____

_____

_____

In Motivational Interviewing, you learned that there are simple and complex reflections. Diving deeper into the complexity of Jerome's situation can help you learn more about his conflict or struggle. Here are seven complex reflections to let him know you remain an attentive listener and understand the deeper issue.

Double-sided reflection is when you present both sides of a problem. You might say, "On one hand, the pain in your stomach makes you not want to eat. On the other hand, it has been a long time since you had a meal."

Affective reflection is pulling out the emotion you heard. You might say, "You feel more open to trying stuff."

The metaphor is using an analogy to reflect a point. You might say, "Your hunger is causing you to starve to death."

Continuing Paragraph reflection is when you are guessing what someone is feeling. You might say, "And you now think that this pain is hunger."

Emphasizing Personal Choice is about promoting autonomy. You might say, "Now you can decide if this is hunger or not."

Amplification is when you emphasize a stated behavior. To Jerome, you might say, "Not eating doesn't cause any problems."

Siding with the Negative is similar to Amplification. Removing choice, but siding with the inability to change a situation prompts the listener to take the opposite position, which could effect change. You could say, "You know you can't make your stomach pain go away."

FEELING STUCK

Pause for a moment, and identify whether feeling stuck is Pleasant, Neutral, or Unpleasant. Regardless of your answer, feeling stuck may invite the Monkey Mind to start chattering, or for you to jump into the "time machine," moving from the past to the future to try to stop this feeling. The mind is ping-ponging: What do I need? What about their needs? How can I satisfy them all? What is the solution?

The Mindfulness solution is that when you become stuck, you will choose curiosity over critical, rash, or reactionary options.

The ability to become curious is a skill that will grow and become second nature with practice. With curiosity, you can open the mind to seeking not the "right" answer, but the self-compassionate choice by asking, "What is the kind thing to do in this situation?" Shifting away from what is "right" can help you identify the ambivalence or the conflict of the situation. When you can clearly see the struggle, you are often better able to identify the choices that ARE available, instead of the choice you think you "should" do, or the simple choices you "crave," or the choice that ignores your needs.

SELF-COMPASSION, FEELINGS, AND NEEDS

Now that you have reviewed the concept of self-compassion, you will want to consider how it relates to your feelings and your needs. Once again, your feelings and needs are tied in an impressive knot together. The good news is that your feelings, which you learned how to observe in Step 2, can provide you with clues about your needs and that your needs may help you better understand your feelings.

CONNECTING

When I was going through my divorce, I remember feeling overwhelmed. My friend looked at me and asked, "Megrette, have you thought about what you need?" I remember the thousand pounds of fear in the pit of my stomach. I looked at her and said, "I can't go there right now." I was terrified at that moment. I couldn't think of anything scarier than my having to sit with my feelings to learn what I needed. I was grateful when she just smiled and gave me three tools, discussed in Chapter 5: Permission, Freedom, and Space. These tools later helped me sit with the angry bull in my mind and gave me the courage to think about my needs.

EXPLORING NEEDS

At this point, it is clear that the quality of your feelings seems to be related to your needs. Feelings that are sharp and unpleasant likely indicate that your needs have not been met, while feelings that are welcoming and soft indicate that many of your needs have been met.

COUNSELING ACTIVITY – **MEETING YOUR NEEDS**

In this section, you are going to look closer at your needs. In the appendix is the handout *A List of Needs*. This list is not exhaustive, but it is a starting place for exploring needs. Using *A List of Needs* and a highlighter, identify the needs that resonate with you. Needs are shaped by your life experience and are derived from your beliefs and values. Your needs and your feelings overlap. Your needs, like a growing child, are in a state of flux, dynamic and always changing. Exploring your needs is an ongoing process, supported by the contemplative practices described in Chapter 4 — meditation, yoga, journaling, or storytelling. Continue to resist judging your needs, which can lead to shame, blame, or guilt. As you have learned, it remains more effective to observe, evaluate, or categorize them.

Begin by noticing the frequency of some feelings. For example, Jerome noted that he was annoyed that people kept telling him that he was feeling was hunger. What need did Jerome have that wasn't being met? Look at *A List of Needs*, and see whether one pops out for you. Did you choose autonomy or space? Maybe what Jerome needed was some time to figure it out for himself.

Evaluating your needs can help you decide between two points. You can ask, "Is this a need or a craving?" Look at *Image 11*, to help you choose between options.

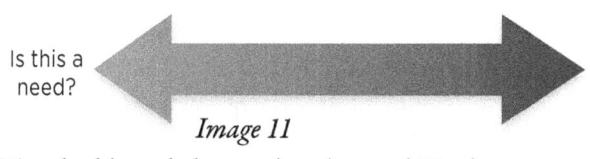

Image 11

This double-ended arrow has the word Need on one side, and Craving on the other.

Mindful Eating recognizes that this evaluation is made easier by bringing in a level of self-compassion and asking, "How can I help myself?" Your needs and desires are complex, and you don't have to rush or feel pressured to meet them. However, when your needs/desires are not being met, they keep returning, often stronger than they were before. As you have learned, not getting your needs met can make you a bit cranky. Mindfulness can help you see a pattern. Try to see your needs and desires as two helpful emotional states that work together to provide both motivation and direction. By asking questions such as, "What do I need?" and "What do I desire?" you have paused and brought curiosity and the spotlight of attention to a typically difficult situation. This decision is filled with merit!

Now on the other side of the arrow is craving. Craving often feels urgent, and this sense of "NOW" can ensnare your better judgment. A pause can give your cravings space to provide you with more options. Cravings are often described as hooks that catch you and prevent you from using your inner wisdom. They are also thought of as "sticky" and cling to your thoughts, actions, and behaviors.

Needs and cravings are grouped together but they are very different. One way of thinking about needs and cravings is to imagine that you are driving and you see a white cloud ahead. You slow down and wonder, "Is that fog or smoke?" Fog can make it hard to see ahead, but when it lifts, there is no lingering trace of it. The smell of smoke, on the other hand, will cling to your clothes, and even though it can't been seen, you still smell it, and feel the sticky residue it leaves behind. Finding yourself in the middle of fog or smoke requires you to take extra care. Thick fog can make it hard to see. Smoke can often indicate danger is present (or in my case that dinner is done!). The Meeting Your Needs Arrow is trying to help you pause and determine, "is this fog (a need) or smoke (a craving)."

GOING DEEPER
Debrief the Meeting Your Needs Activity

1. Take a moment and write down what you or your client liked about using the Meeting Your Needs Arrow.

2. What didn't you like about the activity? How would you change it to better meet your needs?

3. Stretch your skills by spending some time in reflection. Ask yourself the following three questions:

- How have I seen this concept of meeting my needs presented?
- Can I convey the concept of meeting our needs in my own words so it is authentic to me and my clients?
- What opportunities can I seek from clients or more experienced professionals to advance my counseling skills?

REDUCING NEGATIVE EXPERIENCES

Step 3 of the Mindful Eating Map includes mini-steps. Step 3b asks you to describe ways to reduce the negative experience associated with your unmet needs. Use your observation skills: What choices do you see? Step 3c connects you to the self-compassion of Mindful Eating. "Dig even deeper, and add a level of self-compassion to your evaluation. What opportunities exist for you to meet your physical, emotional, and social needs in a way that does not cause harm to yourself or others?" In Chapter 3, you learned about the three parts of self-compassion: Self-kindness, Common Humanity, and Mindfulness. Step 3c asks you to bring an aspect of self-compassion into your decision-making process.

Changing your experience depends on your ability to observe the present moment. As the saying goes, *The past cannot be changed, and the future hasn't come. The present moment is the only time when a choice is possible.* In Chapter 9, you will learn how to create a Mindfulness counseling practice. Until then, keep exploring and playing with Steps 1 through 3 in the Mindful Eating Map.

MAKING DECISIONS TO MEET YOUR NEEDS

Once you understand your needs, meeting them is easier. Remember back in Section One, Chapter 3, where you learned about the three components of self-compassion: Self-Kindness, Common Humanity, and Mindfulness?

The delight of Mindful Eating is you have become self-compassionate in making your food choices. Bringing self-compassion to food and eating makes Mindful Eating different from other programs. Imagine the three parts of self-compassion as questions to reflect on, which will help you connect what you know in your mind to what you know inside, a.k.a. your "inner wisdom." Accessing your inner wisdom will provide valuable information for choices, decisions, and conflicts. Self-compassion isn't an absolute, like judgmental thoughts and thinking. It is on a continuum. One end of the scale is the question: What is the kind thing for me to do for myself? On the other end of the scale is the question: What is the kind thing for me to do for my fellow man?

Right away, you can see an ethical dilemma. "Do I do what is kind for me or what is kind for someone else?" This question may create a feeling of ambivalence or even fear. It is infrequent that you can do both — meet your needs and the needs of your fellows. The inability to "do it all" creates the feeling of being unsure or stuck, which, you might guess, is a big reason people stop eating mindfully.

USING A COMPASSION ARROW

Many times, clients get stuck because there isn't a clear answer. They understand and want to change, but they just aren't sure what to do. If this is happening, consider using the Compassion Arrow, which is depicted in *Image 12* below. The Compassion Arrow is similar to The Meeting Your Needs Arrow, however, the goal is to identify the compassionate choice. On one end of the double-sided arrow is the question, "What is the kind thing for me to do for myself?" On the other side: "What is the kind thing for me to do for my fellow man?" These two questions present the two extremes. They typically will generate great discussion and opportunities to clarify the motives and desires that are present in a session. You can refer back to the Motivational Interviewing skill of DARN, which signals that a client wants to change. Using EARS will help you clarify the importance of and build motivation for changing. In Mindful Eating, the question between the two extremes is, "What is the kind thing to do in THIS situation?" Adding in this level of kindness is a question that may have been overlooked by the client.

JEROME'S COMPASSION ARROW

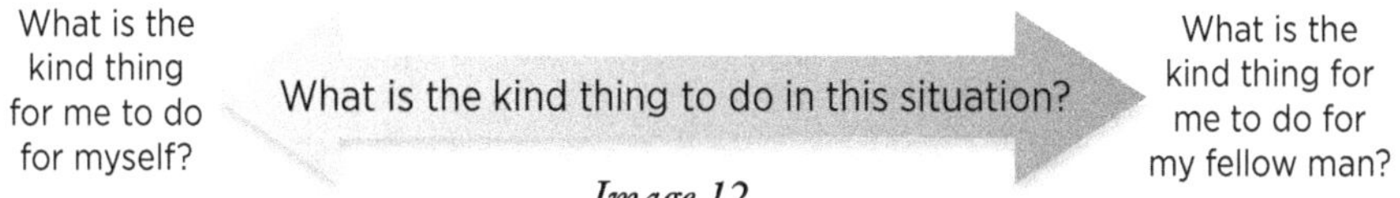

Re-read Jerome's comment in the activity Exploring Feeling Using Complex Reflections. You decide to use the Compassion Arrow with Jerome.

What is the kind thing for me to do for myself? ← What is the kind thing to do in this situation? → What is the kind thing for me to do for my fellow man?

Image 12

You say to him: "Jerome, what is the kind thing to do in this situation?" He replies with a shrug. You hand him a Compassion Arrow and you offer, "I am concerned that your needs are not being met." Ask him, "What would be a kind thing for you to do to help yourself?"

- What does Jerome say?

Then you ask, "What would be a kind thing to do for other people you are with?"

- What does Jerome say?

Finally you ask Jerome, "What is the kind thing to do in this situation?"

- What does Jerome say?

Using the awareness of your feelings and how these related to your needs did the Compassion Arrow shift your counseling session, allowing you to become more resilient when a client gets stuck? The more you clarify the spoken need and listen for the unspoken need, the more empathy and understanding you will develop.

GOING DEEPER
Debriefing the Compassion Arrow

1. Take a moment and write down what you liked about using the Compassion Arrow.

2. What didn't you like about the tool?

3. Stretch your skills by spending some time in reflection. Ask yourself the following four questions:

- How have I observed compassion and self-kindness presented?

- How can I convey self-kindness and self-compassion using my own words and experiences?

- Where can I find an opportunity to observe this concept being taught?

- How can I use this concept to deepen my own counseling skills?

COUNSELING ACTIVITY – **THOUGHT COMPASS ON NEEDS**

Consider whether you would like to complete a Thought Compass of this chapter regarding your needs. If you do not remember the instructions for Thought Compass, go to Chapter 1.

CHAPTER SUMMARY
Identifying Your Needs

HOORAY! Review the counseling tools you just learned.

- Your brain (the physical organ) has seven needs: Sleep Time, Physical Time, Focus Time, Time-in, Downtime, Play Time, Connecting Time.

- An inventory of your feelings can help you understand your needs.

- *A List of Needs* from the Center for Nonviolent Communication has been provided in the appendix.

- Focusing only on the needs of other people is not self-kindness and will not help you change.

- Use the Compassion Arrow to help you identify choice.

- Apply your skills of self-compassion when identifying your needs.

OOPS! Review the struggles you might encounter.

- Identifying your needs starts with observing your feelings.

- Feelings you identify as pleasant likely indicate that your needs are being met.

- Feelings you identify as unpleasant likely indicate that your needs are not being met.

- Tolerating your feelings is an important skill that can guide you to understanding and exploring your needs.

- It is not possible to always meet your needs, which makes self-kindness a necessary part of the evaluation.

TADA! Review the action steps of the chapter.

- Identify your physical needs using the Healthy Mind Platter.

- Engage in nonjudgmental observation of the current situation.

- Identify whether the current situation is Pleasant, Neutral, or Unpleasant.

- Engage in nonjudgmental observation of your sensory, thought, and emotional experiences.

- Review A List of Feelings to help guide you to your needs.

- Identify your needs with self-compassion.

- Create a Thought Compass to help you organize and observe your learning about this chapter.

EMPATHIZING - DAVID

"Yesterday my legs just wouldn't work. I went to a party, which was nice, but I was struggling and totally wiped out afterward. I didn't eat much."

[You have expressed a desire to eat more, so can you tell me more about this choice to not eat?]

[Client looks away from the counselor.]

"I was frustrated. I couldn't seem to get food from the buffet, and then walked back to my chair. I would have had to use my cane and carry both my plate and my drink. Yesterday, I just snacked and had a few drinks."

[Beer?]

"Yeah, I opened the bottle when I was in my chair. It was the easiest thing to take and not spill."

— David

Chapter 8
Creating Your Intention

"Each decision we make, each action we take, is born out of an intention."
— Sharon Salzberg, O Magazine, "The Power of Intention," January 2004

What is an intention? In Mindfulness and Buddhist writings, intention is defined as the exertion of your will to change. There are different types. Described as the "Right Intention"[42] is the desire to give up doing things that cause harm, the desire to generate good will, and the desire to reduce harm. It is easy to get stuck on the word "right," yet I encourage you to hear it as simply a way to harness the positive energy necessary to change. Those intentions that describe an outcome that causes harm or suffering, or that cultivate harmful states, either emotional, mental, or physical, are considered the "Wrong Intentions."

WHY IS POSITIVE ENERGY MORE EFFECTIVE FOR A CHANGE?

Often, the energy driving changes with food and eating is fear or discomfort. As you learned in the introduction to this book, pain, discomfort, and inability are what compel you (and others) to seek help. As you become aware of your pain or discomfort, you begin to make changes to make a situation more tolerable. This is as much logic as it is instinct, because who wants to be in pain? Small changes and tiny tweaks are quick Band-Aids that help you keep going. Unfortunately, they can also cover up the problem and keep you ignoring the underlying cause of it.

The moment you move out of discomfort, the urgency shifts, and your motivation decreases. With pain present, the motivation waves peak, as BJ Fogg, PhD, says: "You have the motivation to do hard things. But it is temporary!"[43] What goes up must come down!

REFLECTING

In a society that has become distracted by the quick fix, it is easy to forget to look beyond immediate relief. Think about what David said in the Empathizing section. His goal was to eat a healthier diet and to stop losing weight. But his immediate frustration with his disability distracted him from this larger goal.

INTENTION HELPS YOU SEE BEYOND THE QUICK FIX

Mindfulness and Mindful Eating offer benefits because they help you process information and use this information to guide decisions. However, there is a space between gathering the information and processing it to help you take action. Here you can empathize with David's struggle feeling helpless at a party, not wanting to ask for help, and learning how he can reduce the harm he feels he is causing himself. I am going to guess here, but I suspect David was angry with his physical limitation and his unmet need of getting nutrition.

Each person is looking to reduce the harm and suffering that he or she is experiencing. This desire means everyone is looking for a solution. However, if the solution is a quick fix and works only for a short time, then it really isn't a solution. In Buddhist teaching, these "quick fixes" are called poisons. Refer to Figure 3: The Three Poisons

Every day, each person in the world unknowingly takes a sip of any or all of the three poisons – unknowing/ignorance, self-destruction/hatred, and craving/greed — hoping that it will help them suffer less, help others, and make everyone happier. Some people take a tiny sip, other people guzzle gallons, all with the same desire — to suffer less, to help others, and to be happier! After days, weeks, years, decades, you may "wake up" and realize the poisons don't work! In time, you realize that what you thought was a cure was really the cause of the problem.

THE THREE POISONS

UNKNOWING/IGNORANCE/DELUSION

Buddhism talks about the poison of "Delusion," which is a strong word and refers to two problems. The first is our incomplete understanding of Reality. No one wants to think that he or she is deluded, but at the same time, few people would claim to know how the whole world works! It is not hard to admit that, as a species, humans are limited in their understanding and knowledge of the world. Everyone struggles to understand the nature of things as they are, free of perceptual distortions.

The second problem is being unaware, or ignorant, of our inner needs. This is not a lack of knowledge — for example, like the lack of knowing how to bake a souffle — but the failure to understand the feelings and experiences within you. Not knowing can be difficult and scary. It takes a great act of courage to admit you want to learn, so if you have taken this step, congratulations! Yet, too often, fear of being unaware can create a cycle of constant searching outside of yourself for happiness, satisfaction, and a solution to life's problems. The concept of delusion is complex, but for the purposes of this book, it is limited to your understanding that the most precious knowledge is the balance you achieve by mindfully evaluating your inner or your outer experience.

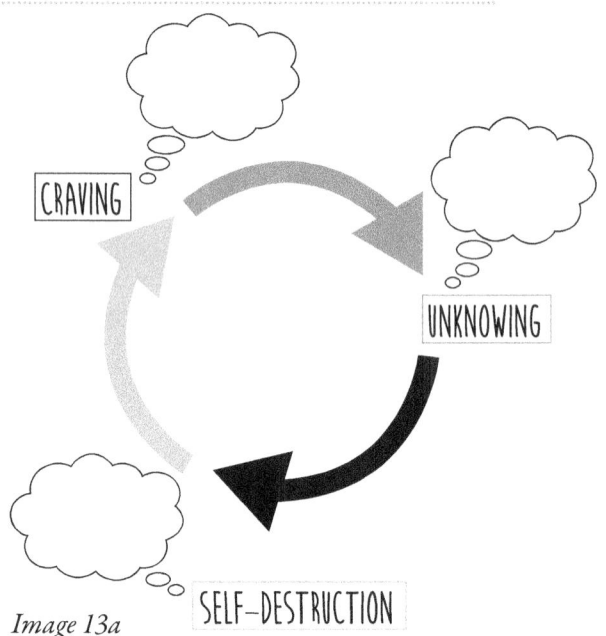

Image 13a

SELF-DESTRUCTION/HATRED

Everyone on the planet has experienced some ill-will or annoyance at something: a rude driver, a frustrating work situation, or unresolved injustice. The symptoms of self-destruction/hatred can show up as anger, hostility, dislike, or ill-will, and wishing harm on another person. This poison might present as aversion, in which you resist, deny, and avoid unpleasant feelings, circumstances, and people. On the other end of the spectrum, it is blinding hatred. You might never experience this extreme, but if the mind is full of hate, a person's thoughts will never be calm, but will be endlessly occupied with strategies of self-protection or revenge. When the poison of self-destruction consumes a person, he or she sees feelings, which are often dark and hard to tolerate, as an internal enemy.

CRAVING/GREED

Recall a moment when you craved something. That burning desire, unquenchable thirst, or lust may seem fresh in your mind. Remember how you wanted this thing to help you feel fulfilled, whole, and complete. The poison of craving and greed is described as an "inner hunger so that we always seem to be striving towards an unattainable goal."[44] This hunger can trick you into thinking that happiness depends on reaching that goal, but once you attain it, you find no lasting satisfaction.

Craving and greed can present as trivial, or they can manifest themselves in compulsive and destructive ways. A sense of being out of control can be reinforced by a person's words, thoughts, and behaviors. Words typically include extremes: never, can't, always, have to, or must. Thoughts reinforce the feeling of being hooked and you can listen for red-flag words such as, "should, have to, not allowed." Craving/greed is just one of the three poisons of an endless and pernicious cycle that brings only suffering and unhappiness.

THE CURE FOR THE THREE POISONS

Mindfulness offers an antidote to these three poisons: nonjudgmental observation, curiosity, and self-kindness. Refer to *Image 13b*.

Overcoming unknowing and ignorance is learned by cultivating curiosity in learning, wisdom, and insight.

Overcoming self-destruction and hatred is learned by cultivating loving-kindness, compassion, patience, and forgiveness.

Overcoming craving/greed is learned by engaging in nonjudgmental observation and to see what is present.

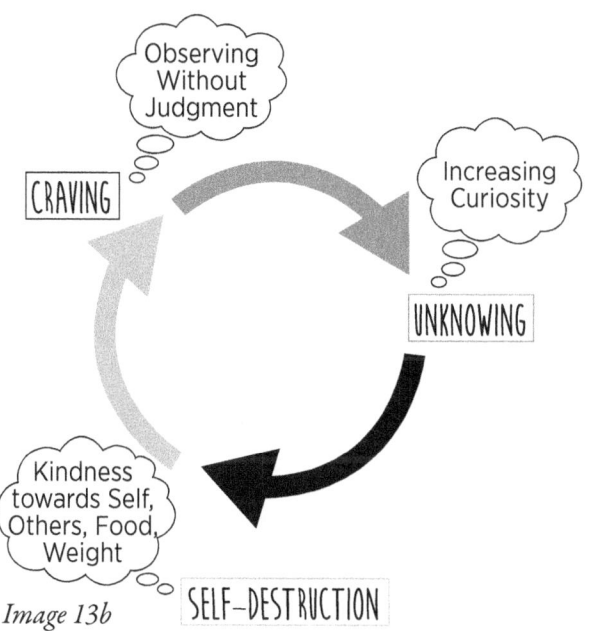

Image 13b

COUNSELING ACTIVITY – CREATING YOUR INTENTION

Ideally, creating and renewing your intentions is woven into your daily contemplative practice. Starting a meditation, prayer, or yoga practice by connecting to your larger intention can help you take smaller sips of the three poisons.

The suggestion can be a formal practice or a simple utterance, such as:

- "May this action reduce the harm I cause myself or others."
- "May this action generate goodwill for myself and others."
- "May this action work to end the suffering in myself and others."

You can bring this intention to all of your actions. For example, when cooking or eating, consider saying:

- "May this meal/food/bite reduce the harm I cause myself or others.
- "May this meal/food/bite generate goodwill for myself and others."
- "May this meal/food/bite work to end the suffering in myself and others."

GOING DEEPER
Debriefing the Three Poisons

1. Take a moment and write down what you liked about the Three Poisons teaching.

2. Ask yourself, Does this teaching ring true to me? If it doesn't, how would you change it to better meet your needs?

3. Stretch your skills by spending some time in reflection. Ask yourself the following four questions:

- Have I observed this teaching before? If so, when?

- Do I wish to I convey this concept using my own words and experiences?

- Do I wish to learn more about this concept? Are there books about Mindfulness that could help me, such as *The Zen of Eating* by Ronna Kabatznick, or *The Buddha's Brain* by Rick Hanson?

- How will I use this information to improve my understanding of Mindful Eating?

HOW IS INTENTION DIFFERENT FROM A GOAL?

The first and most notable difference is that your intention, unlike a goal, is not measurable. Intention is a deep desire to change. While it can be obvious and visible to those around you, it is not easily definable. Articulating your intention to another person can be challenging because it isn't tied to an outcome like weight loss or lower blood pressure. Your intention is not a behavior, but a thought process. When you practice Mindfulness, you are training your mind to think differently, to be aware, to consider your needs and the needs of others in a way that creates less harm. This ethical aspect of Mindfulness and Mindful Eating is linked to your needs – which are linked to your feelings. Your needs and your feelings become entwined, which is a nice way of saying they are all tangled up together, making behavior changes far more complicated than the ad slogan "Just do it."

HOW DOES INTENTION CHANGE YOUR DIET?

One of the most challenging aspects of Mindful Eating is developing nonjudgmental awareness when learning, exploring, and understanding nutrition. The complex and technical science of nutrition seems to promote the idea of a "right" or "wrong" way to eat or that "right" or "wrong" foods exist. Fortunately, the concept of a right or wrong way to eat couldn't be further from the truth.

What is true is that some foods have more nutrients than other foods. Sometimes, your diet feels more balanced than it is in other moments. In some moments, you are more aware, which allows you to better meet your physical, mental and emotional needs. In some moments, eating is more pleasurable than in others. Noticing the frequency of desirable experiences with food, eating, and health, and working toward having more of these experiences, is the intention of Mindful Eating. The intention is never to label your diet or your eating as "right" or "wrong."

I hope you are excited about creating the intention to change your diet and to eat foods that have more nutrients, to focus on finding a new balance of nutrients, to become mindful when eating, and to adapt meals so that eating is a pleasant experience.

Let's learn, or relearn, nutrition in a way to meet these new intentions.

CHOOSING NUTRITION

Referring to *Image 14*, The "Choices" handout, with its five teaching points, was created to assist you. The first point is understanding the concept of choice. When it comes to food and nutrition, having a choice is the first step to Mindful Eating. So many times a situation arises where choice doesn't seem possible. If this happens, pause and remind yourself to "see" the choice. You might simply ask, "What are my options in this moment?"

Once you have identified choice, become aware that each choice is actually two: **Selection and Portion**. What you choose (high-nutrient or low-nutrient food) and how much you choose (of a high-nutrient or low-nutrient food.)

Within these two aspects of choice are four clouds that ask the Mindfulness questions: **Why?** Why that food? Why that amount? As you have already learned, there are many reasons a person would choose a particular food or amount. Mindful observation of senses, thoughts, and feelings help you answer these questions. These observations are **internal**, or information that comes from within you, and **external**, or information that comes from outside of you. Reading through the choices, you might consider your **energy** needs, which is provided by macronutrients, or food with calories. You might also consider the **functioning of your body** as well as **disease prevention**,

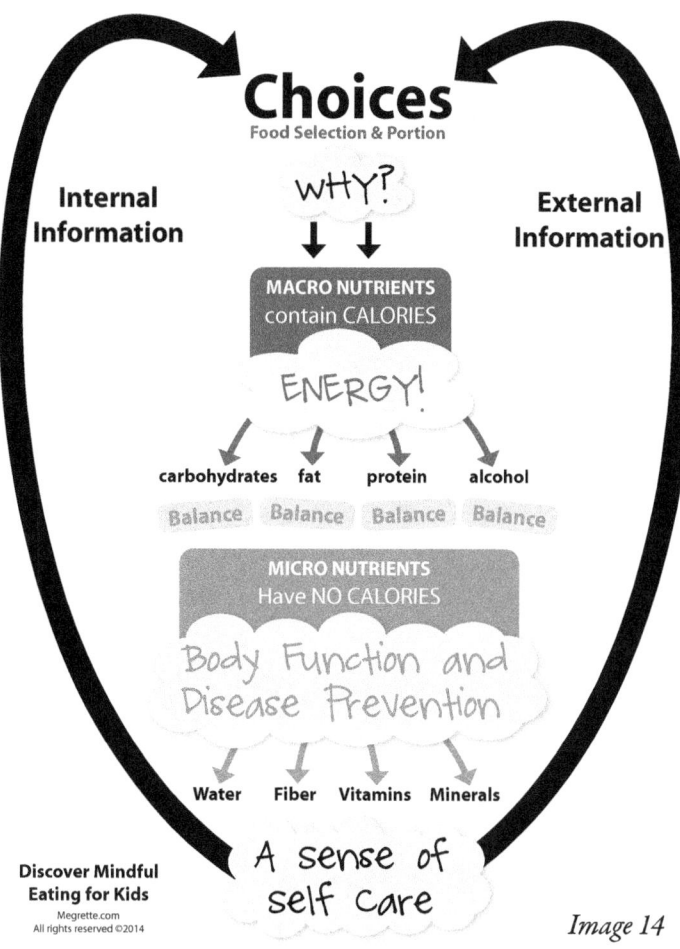

Image 14

which are provided by micronutrients, or substances/phytonutrients that by themselves to not provide calories.

The final intention is for **self-care**. Deciding to make a less-pleasant choice in favor of self-care and self-kindness is how Mindful Eating honors and expresses self-compassion. The act of self-compassion changes your food and eating choices, creating a renewable cycle.

SORTING OUT THE WHYS

You may be unaware how much internal and external information is part of every food decision. By asking "Why?", you can discover whether one choice is more important than another, not because the decision is superior, but to develop awareness, which starts the change process. "Why?" can also help you connect with your intention, your needs, and your feelings. Becoming more aware of these before or while you are eating helps you develop a logical decision-making process.

COUNSELING ACTIVITY – **NICE PANTS!**

You may be thinking, "Yeah but..." and dismissing this approach as something that can't work for you. Let me offer you an activity.

Why did you purchase the pants you are wearing? List all the reasons you bought your clothes. What was the most important reason you chose those pants? Was it cost? If you could find another pair of pants for the same cost, would you buy them? What if they weren't in your size? Are cost AND size important? What if they were in an unattractive fabric? Are cost AND size AND appearance important? What if they were poor quality? Are cost AND size AND appearance AND quality important? What if they didn't fit well? Are cost AND size AND appearance AND quality AND fit important? It is easy to see that you purchase clothes for lots of internal reasons and not just the external reason of cost or availability. When this logic is applied to food, you may be less confident choosing what to eat. This is why Mindful Eating begins with "Why?".

GOING DEEPER
Debriefing the "Nice Pants!" Activity

1. Take a moment and write down what you or your client liked about the "Nice Pants!" activity.

2. What didn't you like about the activity? How would you change it to better meet your needs?

3. Stretch your skills by spending some time in reflection. Ask yourself the following three questions:

- How have I observed the concept of Internal/External factors with food being presented?

- How can I convey this concept using my own words and experiences?

- How can I use the feedback from teaching this concept to deepen my counseling skills?

CONNECTING

Many years ago, I was blessed with an opportunity to take a quilting class from the talented quilter and author Carol Doak. I loved learning how she created so many technical works of art, and I was fascinated by her ability to teach these concepts. Here is how she did it. She would, for example, instruct students: "Place pins across the edge of your fabric, like this." (If you have ever quilted, pinning your work is a necessary step that you wish you could skip!) Then she would say, "Let me show you WHY." She would demonstrate how the seam that was pinned as instructed was superior to the seam that wasn't pinned correctly. For many hours, Carol would demonstrate, then have the students experiment with techniques to determine for themselves which was more effective. This teaching method not only offered autonomy, but also was done without judgment. I remember thinking that anyone who wanted to become a better teacher should take Carol's class, not to learn to quilt, but to learn how to teach technical and tedious skills in a way that was empowering! (The bonus: You will have a beautiful quilt when completed!)

ENERGY

In the "Choices" graphic, the Energy cloud is below the box labeled Macronutrients, which are defined as foods with calories. The four macronutrients are Carbohydrates, Fat, Protein, and Alcohol.

Image 15

0   1   2   3   4   5   6   7   8   9   10

Less energy   **Normal**   **More energy**

Calorie is another word for energy. The body gets hungry to signal the brain that it needs energy. (The subjective and dynamic sensory experience of hunger was discussed in Chapter 4.) When you eat an amount of food that is satisfying, and the balance of macronutrients aligns with your body, you are likely to experience an increase in energy. In Mindful Eating, you can set your intention to become aware of your experience before, during, or after a meal. To determine how you felt after eating, connect to your direct experience. For example, ask yourself, "After lunch, what is my energy level?" Using Figure 4, rate it on the scale of 0-10. Zero represents very low energy, and 10 represents a higher, or more pleasant, energy level.

The funny thing about macronutrients is that you are seeking a balance based on your particular needs at that moment, meaning that eating is a dynamic process that focuses on *balance*, not *perfection*. You have to discover the balance of macronutrients that is ideal for you at each meal. How? In Step 1 of the Mindful Eating Map, you learned to observe your experience, including your sensory information, what you know, and your likes, dislikes, and craving. This step asks you to find the overlap of three sources of information, much like the Venn diagram. Refer to *Image 16*, Balance Point

A phrase that may help you is, "Mindful Eating is about finding the middle way." It is not about find a "perfect" diet or even the notion that a "perfect" diet exists. It is finding a balance that is kind.

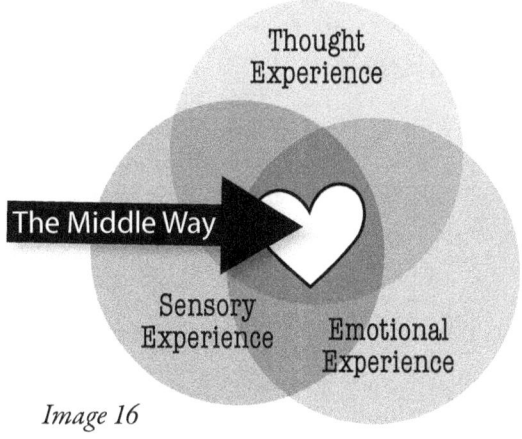

Image 16

BODY FUNCTION AND DISEASE PREVENTION

How well your body functions and its ability to prevent disease are major functions of diet. As science advances, there is more and more understanding of the importance of micronutrients: Water, Fiber, Vitamins, and Minerals.

A simple way to understand these four micronutrients is to consider that water and fiber govern and support body functions — a nice way of saying peeing and pooping. When you experience disruptions in either of these processes, you are having "plumbing problems," such as dehydration, kidney stones, constipation, or diverticulosis. Water and fiber-rich foods support not just peeing and pooping, but also healthy gut bacteria and digestion.

Vitamins and minerals may help the body prevent diseases such as heart ailments, stroke, cancer, and vision loss. By choosing foods that may help to prevent disease, you are investing in your health. For some of you who are working with clients to avoid these health concerns. However as a registered dietitian, you may be working with clients to address the problems where is a more technical process.

Turning back to "Choices," the food you selected will deliver both your energy (macronutrients) and your micronutrients. In 2015, the USDA made a helpful change from recommending nutrient amounts to identifying nutrient-rich foods and suggesting the frequency these foods are consumed. This shift — from getting a designated number of International Units of vitamin A, to eating 4-5 servings per week of red and orange vegetables — makes it easier for you to create an eating plan rich in micronutrients. The decision to talk about food instead of nutrients is to understand that nutrition is about EATING. Research is emerging that how the body digests foods has an effect on how the body absorbs nutrients to nourish the body. In short, new research on the gut is showing that promoting healthy digestion is part of your overall wellness which supports focusing on enjoyment.

WHY NUTRITION GETS CONFUSING

The scientific concept of nutrition may raise questions and confusion. For example, what is the macronutrient difference between white bread and 100% whole-wheat bread? If you look *only* at the macronutrients, there is almost no difference. However, if you look at the micronutrients, 100% whole-wheat bread contains more fiber and vitamins and minerals. This is also true for sweet potato vs. white potato, iceberg lettuce vs. spinach, and so on.

Macronutrients require balancing at each meal, and there are lots of reasons you might change the amount of carbs, fat, and protein. Your energy needs shift depending on your exercise routine, your overall health, and the time of year. (It is true: Your energy needs change with the climate!)

It is also confusing that micronutrients don't provide your cells with energy to function. Micronutrients *assist* the cells with important functions and chemical reactions. Micronutrients may make you feel "well" because the body is functioning better, but they do not fuel the cells. Many people find that eating a micronutrient-rich meal, such as a salad, is great, but they might not feel "filled up" or satisfied. This is because a low-calorie salad is also a low-energy salad!

A SENSE OF SELF-CARE

The practice of self-care is very personal and often, like a tender flower, needs to be protected in the beginning. Praise, encouragement, support, and patience are just as nourishing as the food you select. To help you find a sense of self-care, consider the effort you are spending to help yourself. Refer to *Image 17*: The Effort Scale

COUNSELING ACTIVITY – EVALUATING EFFORT

The Effort Scale depicts three levels of effort. The red section, on the right, represents hard effort; the yellow, in the middle, moderate; and the green section, easy effort. Pause for a moment and ask: Do you feel that your current level of effort is sustainable? Will it help you achieve your larger health goals?

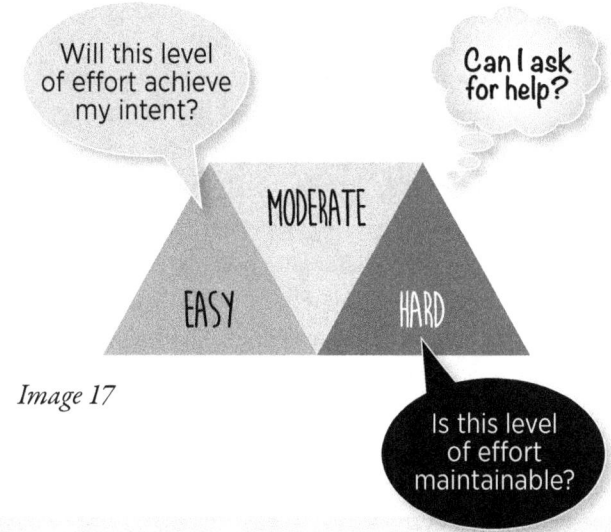

Image 17

GOING DEEPER
Debriefing Choices Activity

1. Take a moment and write down what you liked about the Choices Activity.

2. What didn't you like about the activity. How would you change it to better meet your needs?

3. Stretch your skills by spending some time in reflection. Ask yourself the following four questions:

- Have I observe this concept of choice being presented?

- How can I convey this concept of choice, macro and micronutrients that lead to self-care?

- Do I wish to modify how I teach nutrition to include the concept of choice.

- How can I use the feedback I receive from clients or groups to improve my teaching skills?

GOING DEEPER
Debriefing Evaluating Effort Activity

1. Take a moment and write down what you liked about the Evaluating Effort Activity.

2. What didn't you like about the activity? How would you change it to better meet your needs?

3. Stretch your skills by spending some time in reflection. Ask yourself the following four questions:

- Have I observed the concept of personal effort being presented?

- How can I convey this concept of evaluating effort using my own words and experiences?

- Do I wish to teach this concept in a session, group, or class?

- How can I use the feedback I receive to advance and deepen my counseling skills?

TELL A FRIEND

It is hard to evaluate your effort because you are tempted to think, "if this" or "if that," I *could* do it. However, if your friend said the same thing, you would see her "if this" or "if that" thinking was unrealistic, unreasonable, or unkind. You would tell your friend, "Hey, you don't need to be perfect! Stop making your life so hard. Ease back, go slower, it is OK." Pause and reflect, is there a double standard being presented regarding effort? If you aren't as gentle with yourself as you are with a friend, then re-read self-kindness and self-compassion training in Chapter 3.

Step 4 of the Mindful Eating Map asks that you set your self-compassionate intention to reduce the negative experience associated with your unmet needs. The second part asks that you follow your intention with self-compassion. How? By not overdoing it! If it takes too much effort (i.e., you are in the red zone), you are not likely to follow through with your intentions on a regular and consistent basis! Set your intention to be kind, which includes being kind to your body and offering it food that provides a sense of self-care!

Conclusion

Of all the topics presented in *The Core Concepts of Mindful Eating*, nutrition can be the most challenging. Understanding your intention to explore nutrition without judgment is a huge undertaking and a wide spectrum of information to cover. The topic of nutrition can bring misinformation and hurt feelings, so give yourself encouragement and support. As a Registered Dietitian who practices Mindfulness it is important to keep learning, and talk with other HAES professionals who can share to ways of teaching, advancing your counseling skills. The Center for Mindful Eating offers a list of Mindfulness based counseling programs and trainings to help you advance your practice. You can also use the "Find a Professional" resource to guide your personal needs, and the Good Practice Guidelines can help you find a qualified Mindful Eating teacher.

COUNSELING ACTIVITY – CREATING A THOUGHT COMPASS OF CREATING YOUR INTENTION

Consider whether you would like to complete a Thought Compass of this chapter. If you do not remember the instructions for creating a Thought Compass, go to Chapter 1.

CHAPTER SUMMARY
Creating Your Intention

HOORAY! Review the counseling tools you just learned.

- You know that your intention is not a behavior, but a way of thinking.

- You know that the antidotes to the Three Poisons are curiosity, self-kindness, and nonjudgmental observation.

- The "Choices" handout a Health At Every Size offers a friendly way to explore nutrition.

- The 0-10 rating scale helps you to understand your energy level after eating and to make small changes to macronutrients to meet your energy needs.

- The Effort scale will help you evaluate your effort.

OOPS! Review the struggles you might encounter.

- There is confusion between intention vs. goals. When changing behaviors set and nourish your intention, modify your effort and continue to practice the behaviors that will help you achieve the desired outcome.

- Mindful Eating shifts the focus from a specific food or nutrient to finding balance. This shift can feel abstract and is harder to establish than measurable goals.

- Identifying The Three Poisons: unknowing/ignorance, self-destruction/hatred, and craving/greed in yourself or your client keep

- Evaluate whether you are living in the "red" zone of the effort scale, which is not sustainable over time.

TADA! Review the action steps of the chapter.

- Learn to balance your nutritional needs so you experience improved energy, body functioning, and sense of self-care.

- When considering nutrition, start with the question WHY? Why am I making this choice? Why this food or this amount?

- The antidotes for the Three Poisons: increased curiosity, self-kindness, and nonjudgmental observation, are what nourishes intention, and promotes sustainable change.

- When stuck, identify your needs, with self-compassion. Remember the option of use the Meeting Your Needs Arrow or Compassion Arrow discussed in Chapter 7.

- Set your intention to reduce your unmet needs.

- Create a Thought Compass to help you observe your thoughts.

EMPATHIZING - LINDA

"I love the idea of mindful eating and I really want to bring this into my life fully. I am just not sure how? I try different things and make plans and I always stop. I want to be healthier and to eat healthier but I just don't know how. I mean, that isn't quite right. I know what to do, I just don't know how to keep doing it."

— Linda

CHAPTER 9
Advocating for Your Practice

"You realize that, sure, this setback was hard, but you can deal with it. The ability to eat more mindfully does not automatically make darker thoughts and difficult problems disappear. The ability to eat mindfully helps you accept these thoughts and problems and to continue to 'get up' even when they are present."

— MEGRETTE FLETCHER, M.ED., RD, CDE, "The Fourth Step," Food for Thought

Many people think of calendars as a tool for scheduling events, meetings, or deadlines, but Stephen Covey, author of *The 7 Habits of Highly Effective People*, thinks differently. He was a strong advocate of scheduling self-care time, which he called "Sharpening the Saw." If your saw isn't sharp, work can be harder.

At the heart of Mindful Eating is self-care, which is why in Step 5 of the Mindful Eating Map, you are asked to advocate for your Mindful Eating practice. Only you know what you need or how to care for you. Unless you advocate for yourself — scheduling time for meditation and reflection and to purchase, cook, and savor your meals — these activities will not happen.

CARNEGIE HALL

The skill of planning comes easily for some and is hard for others. Here is a tool to help you create an effective plan. The secret of this tool can be remembered by a famous joke.

> *A woman who was lost in New York City stopped a passerby and asked, "Excuse me. How do I get to Carnegie Hall?" The New Yorker looked at her and said, "Practice, Practice, Practice!"*

The first step in effective planning is to shift your thinking from "doing a behavior" or "completing a behavior" to **practicing** a behavior. The Practice Planning Worksheet is designed to guide your thinking to make this shift.

COUNSELING ACTIVITY – **USING THE PRACTICE PLANNING WORKSHEET**

Practice something, and over time, you will get better at doing it. The Practice Planning Worksheet, or PPW, is an activity sheet that moves you from a Mindfulness activity to a more concrete way to change behaviors, a copy of the Practice Planning Worksheet is in the appendix. If you are interested in only using Mindfulness, focus on the first section (unboxed). This is the most critical part of the worksheet because it helps you identify the behaviors you wish to change.

The second section (boxed) serves as a tracking form. Tracking your "success," or change, can be a double-edged sword. It can help you, but it can wound you at the same time. If it becomes a way to beat yourself up, keep in mind that the intention of the second section is to be helpful, but it is not a critical part of the planning process.

SECTION 1
What to Practice?

In the first section, identify behaviors that you want to practice.

Write down the intention, or the "big" idea, thought, goal, or wish you have. For example:

I want to practice being healthier.

I want to practice eating healthier.

I want to practice being less stressed.

I want to practice eating less after dinner.

I want to practice eating at more regular times.

I want to practice staying hydrated.

These "big" ideas are intentions, which you learned in Chapter 8 will help you see the biggest goal of all, self-care.

THE DEFINITION OF SUCCESS

In this section, you will create your plan to define exactly what you're going to practice. For example, what is your "intention" when you practice being healthier or having less stress? You know that being healthy is not limited to eating, so you include noneating behaviors.

Some examples of "intention":

- You want to practice being healthier. —> Walking is **HOW** you are going to be healthier.
- You want to practice eating healthier. —> Eating less-processed foods is **HOW** you are going to eat healthier.
- You want to practice being less stressed —> Meditating is **HOW** you are going to reduce your stress.
- You want to practice eating less. —> Rating your hunger before eating is **HOW** you are going to eat less.
- You want to practice eating at more regular times. —> Eating 3 meals a day is **HOW** you will eat at more regular times.
- You want to practice staying hydrated. —> Drinking water at meals is **HOW** you are going to improve your fluid intake.

The PPW helps you move from "big" thoughts and aspirations that are difficult to measure to specific behaviors and a plan that can be tracked.

It might be helpful to simply ask yourself, "HOW am I going to achieve this larger intention?" For the PPW to work, you need to think of BEHAVIORS, not outcomes. Behaviors are what you will DO. Outcomes — like weight change, lower cholesterol levels, lower blood pressure — are the results of these changes. The PPW works if you can think of behaviors to change every day. For example, going to the gym once a week or engaging in a monthly breast self-exam would not work well on the PPW.

SECTION 2
Tracking Intention

The next part of completing the PPW is tracking intention. To do this, the PPW uses four numbers:

- **Number 3** represents the BEST you can do when you practice. Write down a reasonable level to shoot for — not a level that can only happen when there is a cosmic alignment of the heavens and you have just won the lottery. Level 3 is not about perfection, which does not exist except in your mind. Instead, choose an ideal standard, an A grade, or the yellow effort level. Ask, is your best effort reasonable? It is a level that will require some effort, but not so much that you don't want to do it the next day.

- **Number 2** is good but not your best. This level represents solid work. It takes less effort, and #2 is a great level when you are dealing with deadlines, or if your attention is focused on other things like work, home, or family.

- **Number 1** is some effort. This represents a bite-size amount of solid work. It might be the effort needed to test blood sugar, to take that 10-minute walk at lunch because you didn't have time in the morning, or to choose to order the side salad so you can say, "I did eat one vegetable!" Think of a number 1 as the level of effort that will "keep the habit alive."

- **Number 0** represents no effort. Maybe you forgot, got busy, or needed to focus on another task. Zero is the rest. It is the time when you need a break or a day off. Please note, you ALWAYS HAVE TO HAVE ZERO in your PPW.

An additional point: Zero does not mean you have lost the desire to change. It means that, on this specific day, you are not moving forward with practicing this desired behavior. Additionally, doing nothing is not the same as harming yourself. This level has no malice or harm associated with it.

Here are some examples of how to complete the PPW.

You want to practice being healthier. —> Walking is HOW you are going to be healthier.

This intention isn't to punish your body, or to engage in extreme workouts. Tracking your intention is defined as walking more, and below is an example of how that might look.

3: 30 minutes of walking is the best.

2: 20 minutes of walking is good.

1: 10 minutes of walking is some effort.

0: 0 minutes of walking will happen when plans change.

You want to practice eating healthier —> Less-processed foods is HOW you are going to eat healthier. Track your intention, which isn't to restrict or deprive. In this example, it is to choose less-processed foods.

3: 1 processed food a day.

2: 2-3 processed foods a day.

1: 4-5 processed foods a day.

0: Didn't keep track.

You want to practice being less stressed —> Meditating is HOW you are going to reduce your stress. You are not better if you meditate longer. You are just establishing an intention to sit.

3: 15 minutes of meditation a day.
2: 10 minutes of meditation a day.
1: 5 minutes of meditation a day.
0: 0 minutes of meditation that day.

If this is not clear, you are welcome to fill out the worksheet and experiment. Use a pencil, and **erase** if you don't like what you are practicing. It is not a test; you can change it anytime you want. Honest.

Practice Planning Worksheet

EVALUATE YOUR RESULTS

So, you completed your first Mindful Eating activity. Congratulations! This is the point where you can evaluate change! Here is a snap-shot of the PPW. Below tracking your intention are the days of the week. Below each day, record how you did on each of the activities you wanted to practice.

day	Tuesday	Wednesday	Thursday	Friday	Saturday	Sunday
ce #1=	Practice #1=	Practice #1= 2	Practice #1= 1	Practice #1= 1	Practice #1= 2	Practice #1= 3
ce #2=	Practice #2=	Practice #2= 0	Practice #2= 0	Practice #2= 3	Practice #2= 2	Practice #2= 3
ce #3=	Practice #3=	Practice #3= 3	Practice #3= 2	Practice #3= 3	Practice #3= 1	Practice #3= 2
		5	3	7	5	8

This is where you evaluate how each activity went. For example, say on Wednesday, you were busy and forgot to "check in and see if hunger was present" before eating.

For Wednesday, on Practice #2, you would record 0. Repeat the process, evaluate how you did for each practice, and record your results.

This should take no more than 15 seconds, which is a very short amount of time!

We all learn differently, so for those of us who are visual learners (myself included), I have included a graph.

GOING DEEPER
Debriefing the Practice Planning Worksheet Activity

1. Take a moment and write down what you or your client liked about the Practice Planning Worksheet?
2. What didn't you like about the activity? How would you change it to better meet your needs?
3. Stretch your skills by spending some time in reflection. Ask yourself the following four questions:

- How have I observed the concept being presented of practicing a behavior?
- How can I convey this concept using my own words and experiences?
- Have I had an opportunity to review other ways to change behavior?
- How will I use the feedback I have received from establishing a clear intention plan to deepen my counseling skills?

WHY ADVOCATING ETHICALLY?

What are the ethics of Mindful Eating? The practice has no lists directing you to eat this, don't eat that, give up meat, eat organic, or stop buying processed food. To advocate ethically is a decision-making process that is personal and unique to you.

THE HEALTH IMPACT

The impact that food has on the health of living beings is obvious. Harm can derive from not eating, from eating too much, from eating foods that hurt other living beings, from the environment, the climate, and the earth itself. Food's huge impact on health comes from the underlying need to eat. Food, eating, health is woven into your culture, into cultures around the world, magnified each day by the choices made by billions of people.

Understanding the ethics of eating is a process that you may struggle with. Several models can assist you, including the definition of self-compassion in Chapter 3. How you choose to view the ethics of food and eating will depend on your needs and values, and it is likely that your ethics will change many times during your life.

THE ENVIRONMENTAL IMPACT

Things to consider include the report of the 2015 Dietary Guidelines Advisory Committee for the U.S Department of Agriculture recommending that Americans consider the environmental impact of their food choices. The committee agreed that there was strong scientific evidence of the benefits of sustainable-food practices. Unfortunately, these recommendations were not included in the final 2015 USDA document.

The committee's work, available for review, is helpful for understanding the scope of this issue. To begin, consider two definitions: What is food security? What is a sustainable diet?

> **What is Food Security?**
> Food security exists when all people, now and in the future, have access to sufficient, safe, and nutritious food to maintain a healthy and active life.

> **What is a Sustainable Diet?**
> Sustainable diets are a pattern of eating that promotes health and well-being and provides food security for the current population while sustaining human and natural resources for future generations.

The USDA committee presented strong evidence recommending that the United States evaluate and consider implementing sustainable food practices. "The environmental impact of food production is considerable," the committee wrote, "and if natural resources such as land, water, and energy are not conserved and managed optimally, they will be strained and potentially lost."[46]

WHY ADVOCATING ETHICALLY IS PERSONAL

Step 5 of the Mindful Eating Map asks you to advocate for yourself and all living beings ethically. The word "ethically" was not added as an afterthought or because it is a "nice" thing to do. Ethics are an important part of your Mindful Eating practice for a reason that may surprise you.

When you choose to act ethically, you are making a choice to see all sides of a situation. When you choose to act ethically, you agree to explore a situation that is often greater than it appears. Ethics are the process of consideration, defined as "moral principles that govern a person's or group's behavior."[47] Your ethics are tied to every part of your being, from your past to the future you wish to create, and from knowledge, wisdom, books, and conversations. It includes your needs, your hopes, your dreams expressed in each moment you are alive. Acting ethically is the decision to care about the whole as well as the parts. When a person chooses to act ethically, a beautiful, compassionate wisdom emerges. While this wisdom is difficult to articulate, poets among us have chosen to try.

ENLIGHTENED PIZZA?

While dining in Burlington, VT, I had the chance to read The Five Faces of Food, panels that hang in the entrance of the American Flatbread Co. Could the ethical struggle that surrounds food and eating be explained by a pizza company?, I wondered. American Flatbread's passion for food is crafted not just in its delicious pizza, but also in an ethical understanding of how people perceive food. Love of food, of eating, of health, of the earth, of the process, is an undeniable force beautifully depicted in the following Five Faces of Food Philosophy. See *Graphic 3-7*.

HUNGER

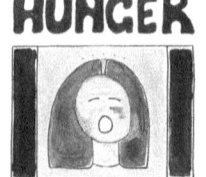

Graphic 3

"I am the face of hunger. I am the first face of food. My body is the great mass and bounty of leaf and flesh. I am hunted and gathered. I am culled and cultivated, cleaned and cured and cooked to fill the emptiness so that the people may rest in peace. This is the first function of food.

"I am the porridge served in Chad and Somalia and Ethiopia and the Sudan. I am the food of prisoners and refugees and the desperate poor of Cairo, Sân Paulo, East St. Louis, and a thousand other places. I am the line between joy and suffering, life and death.

"For those of you who do not stand near this line … be grateful for the kindness of providence, and know this:

"The poor do not hunger out of laziness, but out of circumstance and disadvantage. There is enough food in the world for all. All that remains is to find a way to share it with all." *Graphic 3*

FLAVOR

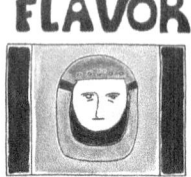

Graphic 4

"I am the second face of food. I am the face of flavor. I am sweet and tart, salt and bitter and fat. I am the miracle of taste and texture.

"I am the warming and the celebration. I am the guide in the wilderness of plants and animals and minerals.

"I speak to the lips and teeth and tongue. I listen to your palate and the depths of your gut for my true voice. And I will guide you toward the food of joy and health." *Graphic 4*

NOURISH

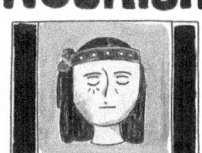

Graphic 5

"I am the third and central face of food. I am the face of nutrition. From my body come the building blocks that give form and strength. I am the fuel that warms the heart and the power to run and dance and dream. I am the purpose of flavor and the way of hunger's pain. Remember me in the foods you eat. I LOVE YOU." *Graphic 5*

NURTURE

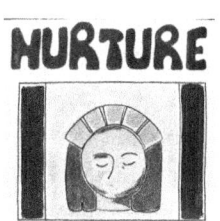

Graphic 6

"I am the face of nurturing. I am the fourth face of food. I am known by the acts of the hands and the heart working together.

"Food that nurtures is grown with care and respect. It is carried without burden and stirred to the songs of kindness. I am the food of the celebration. I am the food of the joy and peace around your table.

"Food that nurtures is shaped by the ways of love. From food made and shared like this flows great happiness." *Graphic 6*

HEAL

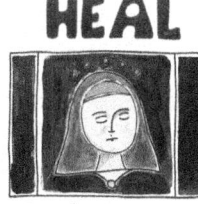

Graphic 7

"Food to fill you. Food of joy. Food for health and comfort. These are the foods of my four sisters. I am the fifth face of food. I am the face of healing. Just as illness and injury take many forms, there are many ways to heal. Food can heal." *Graphic 7*

THE MEMORY OF FOOD

George Schenk, founder of American Flatbread Co., conveys food passion:

> *"The memory of food may seem little more than a mystical contrivance, but not all things that we believe in or hold dear are known empirically. Love is an example. The poets say that love can move mountains, and we see that love is a real force that can change our lives, yet none of us would attempt to quantify it.*
>
> *"Quantum mechanics tells us we cannot observe something without changing it. Our thoughts and acts change our food. And if all of this seems a little hard to comprehend, not to worry, for although science knows quantum mechanics is real, no one truly understands how or why. Like so much of this world and the human condition, food remains as much mystery as measure."*

PRACTICE? DISCIPLINE? DILIGENCE?

Living an ethical life is not easy to do. It often takes practice, discipline, and diligence. These three words are often used interchangeably, but they have very different meanings. You have already explored the concept of **practice**, which focuses not on a specific goal or on getting "good" at something, but on returning to a behavior in a consistent manner. You know that practice differs from a goal, which is a fixed point and, once achieved or accomplished, can be perceived as "done." This sense of completion sheds light on why the change process ends.

You may think you need more **discipline** to achieve a desired outcome. I couldn't agree more, but the word "discipline" comes from the Latin discipulus, meaning pupil or to learn. You do need to learn! We all need to learn — and to keep learning. Discipline is often misunderstood as meaning to punish. Within the concept of discipline is an inherent understanding of **diligence**, meaning persistent work or effort. Neither discipline nor diligence is about punishment. They are about learning from consistent effort. And, yes, everyone will benefit from being diligent when developing a Mindfulness and Mindful Eating practice! Discipline and diligence do not have to be drudgery. In Mindful Eating, as you become aware of your current experience, you are provided with the information needed to make an unpleasant situation better.

One barrier to creating a Mindful Eating practice is a person's inability to effectively evaluate effort, discussed in Chapter 8, or the awareness to not work too hard or too little develops over time. To help you, please refer to *Image 17*, The Effort Scale. By now you know that, despite your best effort, your practice will not be perfect. What should you do when your practice wobbles?

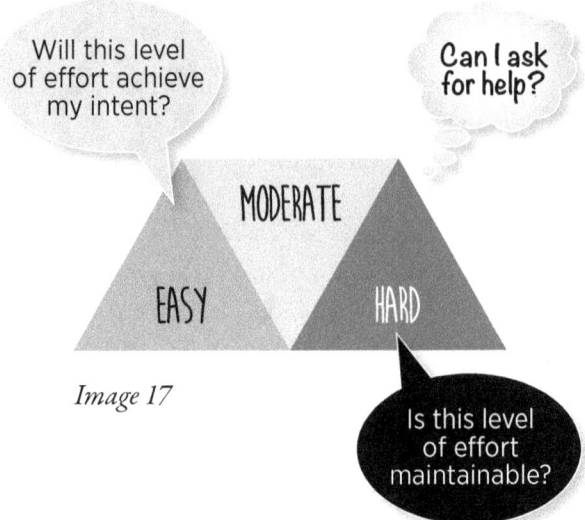

Image 17

OOPS

Stephen Andrew, LCSW, owner of Health Education & Training Institute, teaches this concept, and I have used it at almost all of my classes because it is a joyful way to convey acceptance. Practice "Oops" as a way to forgive and accept your humanness.

DIRECTIONS: Lift your shoulders, maybe raise up your hands, and give yourself a simple "Oops." Once you have said, "Oops," laugh, smile, connect with the common humanity that binds us all together. When you are ready, create a clear intention to avoid re-creating the situation.

RENEWING YOUR MINDFUL EATING PRACTICE

As you can see, creating a Mindful Eating practice is a process of change that is both logical and compassionate, but also strangely complex. This complexity can drain your spirit and motivation. For this reason, The Center for Mindful Eating recommends that you identify ways you can keep your practice alive, or "sharp."

The best way I have found is to be with people who have a similar goal or vision. These are the members of your tribe, your "peeps," your community, or sangha. If you are practicing Mindful Eating, taking a class with a qualified professional will fuel your practice and give it a little lift. If you are committed to the process, consider going on a retreat. If Mindful Eating feels like a practice you want to deepen, attend training from a teacher who has met the Good Practice Guidelines as defined by The Center for Mindful Eating.

CONNECTING

My biggest "Oops" was thinking it would be "easy" to teach Mindful Eating. Boy, oh boy, was I mistaken! Communicating the concept of "being present without judgment when eating" was far from easy or simple or a quick fix! In the early years, I would find myself stuck day after day. Sometimes, it was my ignorance. Other days, it was my arrogance. Each time I got stuck, my craving to talk with other people about Mindful Eating grew.

People ask, "Why did you decide to start the center?" This organization was started after I got so horribly stuck that I HAD to admit, "I was wrong! I need help!" I wasn't able to effectively communicate how to be present, nonjudgmentally, all of the time. When I gathered my courage to speak about this failing, I discovered that everyone was struggling and that I was not alone. You can't imagine the joy I felt when I realized that this desire to be nonjudgmental was hard, not because I lacked some obvious training, but because being present requires more than knowledge. People need practice and support.

What makes The Center for Mindful Eating different is that it was started as a place where you could come and be "wrong," admit your limitations, and discover new options. TCME emerged as a beacon, a light of inspiration to remind all of us, "You are not alone."

How does TCME.org work? When you visit our website, you will discover many free resources for personal and professional use. These resources will get you started on your personal Mindful Eating practice. If you are a professional, you will find the Principles of Mindful Eating and the position statements to guide you.

In the 10 years since The Center for Mindful Eating was formed, it has grown into an international nonprofit that reaches over 100,000 people every year. The Center for Mindful Eating is an alternative to the diet/weight-loss industry. The Center for Mindful Eating, which is member-supported, provides you with more than a place to learn. It offers a wealth of resources, including the Food for Thought newsletter, free professional training, continuing-education credits, handouts, graphical quotes, and much more. If you are not a professional, your individual membership will help ensure that the dark ages of feeling alone and having no place to turn for evidence-based information about Mindful Eating are over!

COUNSELING ACTIVITY – THOUGHT COMPASS ON ADVOCATING FOR YOUR PRACTICE

Consider whether you would like to complete a Thought Compass of this chapter regarding advocating for your practice. If you do not remember the instructions for creating a Thought Compass, go to Chapter 1.

CHAPTER SUMMARY
Advocating for Your Practice

HOORAY! Review the counseling tools you just learned.

- Use the Practice Planning Worksheet to help you establish clear goals.
- Understanding the ethics of Mindful Eating is a personal choice that slowly becomes part of your practice.
- Support your practice by joining organizations that share your values and needs.
- "Oops!" can help you express self-compassion in a fun and funny way.

OOPS! Review the struggles you might encounter.

- Translating your intention into behavior is a new skill.
- Our relationship with food is complex and it ranges from reducing hunger, savoring food, nourishing the body, nurturing relationship, to healing the body!
- The ethics of Mindful Eating may evoke feelings that are difficult to balance with your needs.
- Confusion exists among the concepts of Practice, Discipline, and Diligence.
- It is easy to overdo an activity in a way that is not sustainable.
- Expectations to be "perfect" are unsustainable, and discourage you from evaluating your effort with self-compassion.

TADA! Review the action steps of the chapter.

- Create your goals using the Practice Planning Worksheet.
- Continue to engage in nonjudgmental observation of the current situation.
- Continue to strengthen your formal Mindfulness practice by meditating.
- Strengthen your supports by joining groups that promote the Principles of Mindful Eating.
- Create a Thought Compass to help you identify what you need to advocate for your Mindful Eating practice.

EMPATHIZING - JEROME

"I don't hate coming here anymore. I want to eat a wider variety of foods and to not be so afraid that my mother won't love me. I want to fit in more at school, but it is hard. I feel safer when I don't eat. You are the only person who knows this."

— Jerome

CHAPTER 10
Teaching Your Passion

"I encourage all of you to bring a curious and open mind to each client interaction, and with a growth, rather than outcomes, mindset for your clients."

— SHEILA KELLY, MS, RDN, President, Skelly Skills

The outcome, insight, and connections of learning any subject are unknown. Steve Jobs, creator of Apple, has said his sense of simplicity and design was linked to his taking a calligraphy class in college. J.K. Rowling, author of the Harry Potter series, credits her childhood games for many of the storylines and subplots in her books. There is no single way to help you access your knowledge, inspiration, and motivation.

Throughout this book, you have been encouraged to shift your focus from reaching outcomes, like weight loss or becoming "X," to creating the conditions that will help you live a full and joyful life. The shift from specific to vague can bring frustration, fear, and uncertainty, unless you consider the logic of the shift.

It is true: Life does not come with guarantees. By shifting your focus to creating opportunities for insight and awareness, you increase the probability that it will happen. Think of it this way: You are buying more lottery tickets. Instead of having one chance to nourish your body and whole being, you give yourself two chances, 10, 20, 100, 1,000.

In Mindful Eating, unlike playing the lottery, you engage in behaviors that have merit, such as treating your body with kindness and nourishing yourself with self-compassion, so that even if you don't win some cosmic-enlightenment jackpot, you have still benefited. This is the concept of "merit." It is choosing to create as many "win-win" situations as you can around food and eating. When you shift your thinking from "How can I achieve X?" to "How can I help myself?", something amazing happens. You start helping yourself.

Using mindful awareness, pause and ask yourself: "How can I pave the way for awareness or connections to arise? Can I create a game, offer a project, watch a movie, read or write a poem, share a meal, compare a taste or texture?" Creating the conditions for experiences and experiments to initiate the learning is more effective than only sharing knowledge and facts about nutrition. Experience and experiments help you access your client's unique knowledge. Learning in this way can feel risky because the outcome is uncertain. Teaching in this way does take more time because you are not telling the student what to know, how to feel, or what to think. Yet, you can feel the reward in every moment of teaching — and so can your students.

CREATING ENGAGED LEARNERS

If you are going to teach Mindful Eating, consider using the following four steps: Engage, Theorize, Exercise, Debrief/Relate.

- *Engage the learner.* What would hold your interest? Familiar activities such as writing down what a person ate for the last day or week may feel meaningless and not hold the learner's interest. Let your engagement of the participant support the core emotion you are trying to promote. If the core emotion is curiosity, engage the learner in a curious way. If the core emotions are calm and reflective, what are ways to engage the learner to promote those emotions?

- *Offer a theory.* Put the material in context. Don't feel you have to offer tons of theory or content — many participants already know a lot about the topic. For example, if you are working with patients who are experts in dieting, they likely will need no information about nutrition before beginning an activity.

- *Provide an exercise.* An activity gives participants the opportunity to connect with their direct experience. Don't be fooled: Engaging in an activity is not easy. Learners are typically confused and uncertain. Keep instructions clear and brief. For example, asking a group to break into teams of three can be unsettling and can delay the start of the activity. Instead, have the group count off in threes to establish the smaller groups. For many Mindful Eating activities, check out my two books *Discover Mindful Eating* and *Discover Mindful Eating for Kids*.

- *Debrief/Relate.* Reflect the experience back for the learner. This is when the real learning takes place. Allow adequate time to complete this step. You have already used this concept throughout the book. Let's review how this process might look using *Image 18*: Teaching Theory

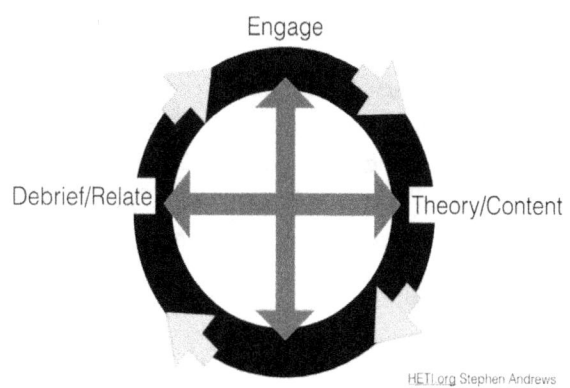

Image 18

Engage: Hi, I would like to ask for your help with my problem of eating past a comfortable level of fullness.

Activity: Could you make a list of all the experiments you have done (or might try) that have helped you learn about the changing sense of fullness?

Debrief/Relate: Thank you. Would you compare your list with mine?

- Rate my fullness before eating.
- Create an intentional pause mid-meal, and evaluate fullness during a meal.
- Rate my fullness after eating.
- Keep a 3-5-day journal of my experience trying to observe fullness.
- Try different meals, and rate fullness level before the next meal.
- Eat the most-enjoyed foods first, saving the least-enjoyed foods for the end of the meal. Reverse this experiment, and evaluate whether there is a difference in eating past a comfortable level of fullness.
- Journal my feelings before eating. After a few days, journal my feelings after eating.

Evaluate whether there were ideas or suggestions worth trying. What are you noticing about the lists? What was most helpful to you and why? What is the idea or suggestion that excites you the least?

Theory: Most people notice that for a person to become aware of their direct knowledge, there is a level of curiosity and personal interest in you, the eater. This curiosity increases when shared in a group or in a pair-share activity. Sharing direct experience is a way to explore and process your life. It helps you create a coherent narrative of your life story. Have participants share their experience. As the Mindful Eating teacher, demonstrate nonjudgment by making clear that experiences are not "good or bad, right or wrong." Evaluate the activity as Pleasant, Neutral, or Unpleasant to help you determine whether it is something to try again. It is a quick way of deciding, "Was this worth it?"

Think about what Jerome said in the Empathizing section preceding this chapter. Do you think traditional nutrition education would have helped Jerome open up and make the connection between his emotions and his food and eating? Do you think using this teaching model, which focuses on activities instead of memorization, is more effective for reluctant students?

GOING DEEPER
Debriefing Engaged Learning

1. Take a moment and write down what you liked about the Engaged Learning Model.

2. What didn't you like about the activity? How would you change it to better meet your needs?

3. Stretch your skills by spending some time in reflection. Ask yourself the following four questions:

- Have I observed this concept being presented?
- Do I wish to use this concept in my teaching?
- If I do, how can I convey this using my own words and experiences?
- Do my sessions have an evaluation to advance my counseling skills?

MAKE LEARNING FUN!

Learning to eat mindfully doesn't have to be difficult, but it may require some detective work. In Chapter 4, you learned to uncover the unspoken desire lurking inside by using Discover, Explore, Play, and Challenge. Consider using yourself as the first student you teach, and experiment with the following phases.

▸ ***Discovering*** what it is you actually desire often requires reflection. Mindful Eating offers so much freedom and choice that you can feel a bit lost without rules and lists of instructions. Reflective techniques described in this book include meditation and the Thought Compass. You can also consult The Tree of Contemplative Practices[48], in Chapter 4. Set aside time for some type of daily contemplative practice, which will help you start the process of listening to your own thoughts, hopes, wishes. and needs. This will help you clarify what you truly desire.

▸ Once you discover what you want, ***Explore*** the options. Say you discovered that Mindful Eating was really an exciting concept. What are ways you can learn more about Mindful Eating? What resources are you aware of? What concepts might overlap Mindful Eating? Some examples:

BodyKindness, Health At Every Size (HAES), sustainable food practices, food security, meditation, self-compassion, acceptance, shame, disordered eating.

▸ After ***Exploring*** your options, you decide to learn more about meditation. ***Playing*** with different types of meditation options can be fun. Let the enjoyment of exploring and learning be part of the Play phase.

▸ ***Challenge***, the last phase, gets you focused on your plan. You are challenging yourself to change. Say you discover you want to stop promoting restrictive eating in your work. What does that desire really mean? You can't just flip a switch and everything is done. It is a process. Start to notice how you feel when you hear restrictive messages at work, in handouts or professional material that you might use for teaching. Refer back to the HAES guidelines to help in your evaluation. As you explore these messages, play with alternatives, conversation comebacks, and other ways to meet your need to move away from teaching and promoting restrictive eating. You may choose to challenge yourself and your colleagues to stop talking about the latest diet or weight-loss attempt. You may choose to challenge your clients to also "give up" restrictive eating.

Remember that noticing your direct experience requires time and attention. With adequate time, the need to rush and be hurried evaporates, creating a sense of space, ease, and opportunity to process life. One of the most helpful parts of Mindful Eating is giving yourself the time to debrief and relate your insights and understanding back to your life. Your insight is the real teacher!

WHERE DO YOU GO FROM HERE?

Books are helpful, but they are not your only teacher. Expand your understanding of Mindful Eating by working with other people, hearing other teachers, and, of course, practicing.

- Phone apps on Mindful Eating, Meditation and Mindfulness are popping up every day. These hand-held tools can offer immediate feedback and support.

- Self-study guides can challenge your learning and understanding. These may use a combination of recorded training and activities for you to try.

- Community support programs, such as online and in-person meditation and Mindful Eating groups, are available.

- Podcasts offer a wonderful opportunity to listen to informative conversations regarding food, eating, change, motivation, and mindfulness. Some examples: *Life Unrestricted; Love, Food; Food Psych; Nutritionally Speaking; The One You Feed; The Art of Authenticity.*

- Web-based learning, available for clients and professionals, can be one-hour lectures or series of lectures and include review of specific books and programs.

- Workshops are typically multiple-day educational events that explore a topic in greater detail and provide practice for honing your skills.

- Retreats, available for clients and professionals, typically run for 3-7 days. Individuals who are committed to Mindful Eating will benefit from participating in longer retreats, often 5-10 days. Retreats provide a chance to immerse yourself in your Mindful Eating practice. Programs such as Green Mountain at Fox Run in Ludlow, VT, offer in-depth residential Mindful Eating opportunities for individuals, where Mindful Eating Conscious Living (MECL) offers a 5-day training for professionals. There are programs at training institutes like Omega, Kripalu Yoga Center, or Aryaloka Buddhist Retreat Center. The Center for Mindful Eating offers a list of professional training programs on its website.

- Meditation instruction, practice sessions, workshops, training, and retreats strengthen your Mindful Eating skills.

The *Good Practice Guidelines*, published by The Center for Mindful Eating, are intended to help you in advancing your personal and professional Mindful Eating practice. These can be found on The Center for Mindful Eating website.

WHAT YOU HAVE LEARNED!

SECTION ONE
The initial section of the book reviewed the three roots for Mindful Eating: nonjudgmental observation, meditation, and self-kindness – the skills needed to start your Mindful Eating journey!

Chapter 1. Your journey started with: What is nonjudgment? Because this is tricky to explain, you were told about the Spirit of Motivational Interviewing, which has four parts: Collaboration, Acceptance, Compassion, and Evocation. These four skills allow nonjudgmental observation to arise naturally. Nonjudgmental awareness allows you to spot shame, which is toxic and will hinder the process of change. You had an opportunity to explore The Principles of Mindful Eating. The chapter ended with the introduction of the Thought Compass, which is a tool to help organize thoughts and ideas.

Chapter 2. Meditation is the foundation of Mindfulness and Mindful Eating. There are many types of meditations. This manual provides you with four types of meditation and two scripts to get you started.

Chapter 3. Self-kindness is part of self-compassion. Mindfulness and Mindful Eating hold the intention for self-kindness in each action, bite, and decision. This rich and emotional concept begins the 13-Inch journey, which is the distance from the head to the heart. There are places where self-kindness are needed: being self-critical, being isolated, and overidentifying. In this chapter, you explored the Motivational Interviewing skill of reflection. You were introduced to the DARN mnemonic and how this relates to putting on your counseling EARS. These two techniques can work together to help identify the motivation and the conflict. You also explored the concept of "merit," which is recognizing the "win-win" situations and behaviors that can help the change process.

SECTION TWO
This marked the shift from basic skills to starting your Mindful Eating journey. Like all great road trips, you need a map — The Mindful Eating Map, a five-step process that was explained in detail in the remaining chapters.

Chapter 4. Sensory experience of Mindful Eating was explored. Learning to apply your nonjudgmental skills and notice your sensory experience provides you with a vast amount of information about yourself. Several helpful tools were provided, such as the Hunger Rating Scale and a way to evaluate your inner experience. The Six Phases of Eating gave you a way to see that eating is a more complex process. You also began the process of balancing your sensory experience with self-compassion and self-kindness, and to explore your inner sensory experience by asking the delightful question, "Is this food Beckoning or Humming for me?"

Chapter 5. Observing your thoughts was the skill of focusing on the thinking process, which, as you learned, can be tricky: It is hard to know that you are thinking! To do this, you explored the value of giving Permission, Freedom, and Space to your Mindful Eating practice. These tools can help you end restrictive thinking, which so often plagues individuals who are skilled and practiced at dieting.

Chapter 6. In the Mindful Eating Map, Step 1 is broken down into three smaller steps. In the step for observing your emotional experience, you were taught how to sit with and nonjudgmentally observe emotions. Because you feel your emotions, there may be a sensory experience associated with them, meaning emotions are not "in your head," but everywhere in your body! As emotions come and go, awareness and self-kindness help you tolerate a spectrum of feelings, allowing you to live a full and rich life. Tolerating your feelings comes from understanding that feelings need not be judged, but can be accepted (even welcomed) as present.

SECTION THREE

This marks the start of applying your direct experience — your senses, thoughts, and emotions — to meet your needs. Not all needs are going to be met, so what do you do? You were provided with tools to increase self-compassion to help ease the experience of unmet needs and to reduce the harm and negative experiences. You explored how to do this for yourself and others, ethically.

Chapter 7. The concept that everyone has needs may be mentally understood, but emotionally, there can be some resistance. In this chapter, you learned how to expand your counseling skills to handle resistance by exploring seven types of complex reflections. You also discovered that learning to observe your needs keeps you on the Mindful Eating path and gives you direction on your Mindful Eating journey. Your needs are on a spectrum, from the physical to the ethical, and your needs are tied to both your feelings and your ability to self-advocate.

Chapter 8. Your intention to change can be derailed by the Three Poisons, which are common actions that seem helpful, but that can trap you in a cycle of suffering. Mindfulness, Knowledge, and Self-compassion are the antidotes to these poisons. Learning how to change your diet mindfully was also reviewed. Using the "Choices" handout, you learned that the intention of Mindful Eating is to find a balance of macronutrients and micronutrients that promotes self-care. Change takes effort, which is why you were given new tools to evaluate your effort so you can create a sustainable practice, changing at a rate that is both compassionate and renewing.

Chapter 9. Advocating for yourself starts becoming clear about your intentions and how you are going to achieve them. This chapter introduced you to the Practice Planning Worksheet. To advocate for yourself and others ethically, you learned the importance of food security and sustainability. These longstanding issues can't be resolved, but are reduced when you consider them as part of your daily eating decisions. The pull to be perfect is within all of us, and thus, the concept of "Oops!" was presented, adding humor and self-compassion to developing the skill of acceptance.

Chapter 10. Teaching your passion is where you are. What is the next step for you? In this chapter, you were presented with a teaching model to guide your discussions and activities. You reviewed the four key words for promoting change: Discover, Explore, Play, and Challenge. These concepts can make a serious conversation lighter, helping you see new opportunities! Finally, this chapter discussed how you will choose to continue your learning. You were introduced to the Good Practice Guidelines and reviewed how to nourish your intention to eat more mindfully by online learning, phone applications, Mindful Eating workshops, retreats, centers, and training programs.

Final Thoughts

*"However mean your life is, meet it and live it;
do not shun it and call it hard names."*
— Henry David Thoreau

It is with gratitude and appreciation that I conclude this book. It is a privilege to join you on the journey of understanding the Core Concepts of Mindful Eating.

Lots of people ask: "Megrette, why do you do this?" Some wonder if I have struggled with food and eating, or if there is some deep-rooted explanation for my passion. Here is what I like to share. I have my demons, my scars, my darker childhood memories, just like you. I have befriended them to the best of my ability. My demons have not disappeared, but they no longer annoy or control me.

And so, the question returns to "Why are you motivated to help?" It wouldn't be possible for me to keep silent and watch you hurt yourself, and it is not possible for me, a registered dietitian and certified diabetes educator, to remain silent and watch the wholesale promotion of the belief in: "Hate yourself happy, healthy, or physically well." You may find, after reading this book, that you agree it is time to stop the suffering caused by hate and to start healing ourselves.

Once you see this suffering, you may be, as I have been, moved to tears. After more than one good cry, you may be motivated to reduce the suffering that touches every aspect of food and eating. If you are, please let me encourage you to join a community of wonderful, passionate people who share your thoughts, beliefs, and passions. These people may be interested in Mindful Eating as The Center for Mindful Eating has defined it, or in helping ease hunger; prevent or treat disease or disordered eating; cook delicious food; or nourish the planet. Regardless of the bonds that connect us, together we can support and nourish the desire to help ease the suffering around food, eating, health, and size acceptance. This craving to help can get confusing, and yes, we can get sidetracked by our own demons. Deep breath. Despite our insights, we will remain remarkably human. If you can let this difference exist and see the common passion, our unique talents will come together and grow stronger. By listening to each other, we can join together and become an army of committed people, professionals, researchers, and food producers who are able to see the big picture and make a dent in the global suffering around food, eating, and health — and have a good, fun, rewarding time in the process!

CHAPTER SUMMARY:
Teaching Your Passion

HOORAY! Review the counseling tools you just learned.

- You have learned a great deal. Congratulations!

- You now have a number of Mindful Eating teaching tools to bring into your everyday counseling sessions.

- You have a clear understanding of The Core Concepts of Mindful Eating.

- You have a clear understanding of the Mindful Eating Map to guide your educational teaching.

- Have FUN!!!

OOPS! Review the struggles you might encounter.

- Engaging your clients is best done by inviting the learner to participate, as described in Chapter 10.

- Many professionals have to change their teaching style to use Mindful Eating and Motivational Interviewing effectively.

- *The Core Concepts of Mindful Eating* is not enough for you to meet the Good Practice Guidelines, as defined by The Center for Mindful Eating, for teaching a Mindful Eating program. Additional training is necessary.

- Remembering Play is how you can avoid getting too earnest and rigid with Mindful Eating. Play can also remind you to check in and see whether your intention is to be perfect. You can't play perfectly! This check can help you keep your intention on fun, enjoyment, and easing suffering in yourself and assisting others to do the same.

TADA! Review the action steps of the chapter.

- Create or adapt your current program to use the Engaged Learning Model.

- Make learning fun! Discover, Explore, Play, and Challenge!

- All of the images, handouts, and activities in this book are available on the Megrette.com website.

A List of Needs

Air	Play	Growth	Respect/ Self-respect
Balance	Recreating	Hope	Security
Comfort	Spontaneity	Learning	Stability
Food	Beauty	Meaning	Support
Nourishment	Communion	Participation	Trust
Physical Well-Being	Ease	Purpose	Warmth
Protection	Equality	Self-Expression	Autonomy
Rest/sleep	Equanimity	Stimulation	Choice
Sexual expression	Harmony	Understanding	Freedom
Safety	Inspiration	Wholeness	Independence
Shelter	Order	Acceptance	Privacy
Sustenance	Peace	Affection	Space
To Thrive	Tranquility	Appreciation	Silence
Touch	Wonder	Belonging	Mourning
Water	Aliveness	Closeness	Discovery
Authenticity	Awareness	Communication	Efficacy
Honesty	Awe	Community	Effectiveness
Integrity	Challenge	Companionship	Intimacy
Presence	Clarity	Compassion	Love
Self-worth	Competence	Connection	Empathy
Transparency	Consciousness	Consideration	Inclusion
Adventure	Contribution	Consistency	Interdependence
Celebration of life	Creativity	Cooperation	Mutuality
Humor	Movement	Exercise	Nurturing
Joy	Laughter		

Image 19

PRACTICE PLANNING WORKSHEET

#1
I want to practice...

Definition of success
3 =
2 =
1 =
0 =

#2
I want to practice...

Definition of success
3 =
2 =
1 =
0 =

#3
I want to practice...

Definition of success
3 =
2 =
1 =
0 =

MONDAY	TUESDAY	WEDNESDAY	THURSDAY	FRIDAY	SATURDAY	SUNDAY
Practice #1 =	*Practice #1* =	*Practice #1* =	*Practice #1* =	*Practice #1* =	*Practice #1* =	*Practice #1* =
Practice #2 =	*Practice #2* =	*Practice #2* =	*Practice #2* =	*Practice #2* =	*Practice #2* =	*Practice #2* =
Practice #3 =	*Practice #3* =	*Practice #3* =	*Practice #3* =	*Practice #3* =	*Practice #3* =	*Practice #3* =
Total =	***Total*** =	***Total*** =	***Total*** =	***Total*** =	***Total*** =	***Total*** =

9. _____
8. _____
7. _____
6. _____
5. _____
4. _____
3. _____
2. _____
1. _____
0. _____

MONDAY	TUESDAY	WEDNESDAY	THURSDAY	FRIDAY	SATURDAY	SUNDAY

Megrette.com
Mindful eating made easy

Hugs, Gratitude, and Thanks

I would like to give thanks to my supports. These include:

My kids, Claire and Jane, who have always been my first students. I give thanks to my family, especially Nick, Sarah, Paul, and Peg. I give a hug to my dog, Bea, who reminded me every day to take a walk. I give thanks for my peers, Sondra, Barbara B, Mary S, Louise, Cheryl, Lori, and Liz B, for their efforts to help me with this book. I give thanks to my friends at WDH and WHP and some extra big hugs to Vicki, Marianne and Kris for the endless encouragements. I give a big hug to David for his ability to make this book beautiful and to Sue my editor for her sharp eyes and wordsmithing.

I would like to give thanks to my teachers. These include:

The past, current, and future board members and staff at The Center for Mindful Eating. Steven and John at HETI for their willingness to teach Motivational Interviewing, and Cheryl for her cheering the MI students to keep going. To Aryaloka Buddhist Retreat Center for offering a place to practice and teach Mindful Eating.

I would like to give thanks to the future Mindful Eating teachers who will be able to demonstrate the value of nonjudgment, compassion, and wisdom.

Training Resources

There are many wonderful programs that can expand and deepen your understanding of how to eat a nourishing diet mindfully. Please visit megrette.com for links to these programs. Here are the programs that I believe are exceptional:

- Continuing Education on Mindful Eating available at The Center for Mindful Eating
- Motivational Interviewing Training
  - Stephen Andrews, LCSW
  - Dawn Clifford PhD, RD
  - Angelina Moore Maia PhD, RD, LD
  - Susan Dopart, MS, RD
  - Dr. Ellen Glovsky, RD, PhD
  - Molly Kellogg, LCSW, RD
- Core Concepts in Mindful Eating Live Training
- Intuitive Eating Training
- Am I Hungry Training
- MECL, Mindful Eating Conscious Living Training
- Eat for Life Training
- MB-EAT, Mindfulness-Based, Eating Awareness Training
- MBSR, Mindfulness-Based Stress-Reduction Training
- ACT, Acceptance and Commitment Training
- NVC, Nonviolent Communication Training
- Self-Compassion Training
- Eating Competency Training

The following are philosophy or position statements:

- The Principles of Mindful Eating
- The Position Statements of The Center for Mindful Eating
- Health At Every Size Community

Visit Megrette.com/coreconcepts for additional resources.

Footnotes

[1] Bacon, Linda, and Lucy Aphramor. "Erratum To: Weight Science: Evaluating the Evidence for a Paradigm Shift." Nutrition Journal 10.1 (2011): n. pag. Web. <https://nutritionj.biomedcentral.com/articles/10.1186/1475-2891-10-9>.

[2] Mann, T; Tomiyama, AJ; Westling, E; Lew, AM; Samuels, B; & Chatman, J. (2007). Medicare's Search for Effective Obesity Treatments: Diets Are Not the Answer. American Psychologist, 62(3), 220 - 233. doi: 10.1037/0003-066X.62.3.220. UCLA: 393158. Retrieved from: https://escholarship.org/uc/item/2811g3r3

[3] Hudnall, Marsha. "Mindful Eating in Nutrition Counseling for Eating Behaviors: What Research Suggests." Today's Dietitian Jan. 2016: n. pag. Web.

[4] A Curious Stance, "Food for Thought Handout Archives 2006-2013." Issuu. The Center for Mindful Eating, n.d. Web)6 Feb. 2017.

[5] Fox, Kieran C.r., Savannah Nijeboer, Matthew L. Dixon, James L. Floman, Melissa Ellamil, Samuel P. Rumak, Peter Sedlmeier, and Kalina Christoff. "Is Meditation Associated with Altered Brain Structure? A Systematic Review and Meta-analysis of Morphometric Neuroimaging in Meditation Practitioners." Neuroscience & Biobehavioral Reviews 43 (2014): 48-73. Web.

[6] Eberth, Juliane, and Peter Sedlmeier. "The Effects of Mindfulness Meditation: A Meta-Analysis." Mindfulness 3.3 (2012): 174-89. Web.

[7] Chen, Kevin W., PhD, MPH, Margaret Chesney, Phd, Susan Gould-Fogerite, Edward Mills, PhD, Karen Sherman, PhD MPH, and Bonnie Tarantino. "Meditation Programs for Psychological Stress and Well-Being." Agency for Healthcare Research and Quality. U.S. National Library of Medicine, 01 Jan. 2014. Web. 06 Feb. 2017.

[8] Crane, C., Barnhofer, T., Duggan, D. S., Hepburn, S., Fennell, M. V., & Williams, J. M. G. (2008). Mindfulness-Based Cognitive Therapy and Self-Discrepancy in Recovered Depressed Patients with a History of Depression and Suicidality, Cognitive Therapy Research, 32, 775–787.

[9] Ivtzan, I., Gardner, H. E., & Smailova, Z., (2011). Mindfulness meditation and curiosity: The contributing factors to wellbeing and the process of closing the self-discrepancy gap. International Journal of Wellbeing,1(3), 316-326.

[10] Higgins, E. (1987). Self-discrepancy: A theory relating self and affect. Psychological Review, 94 (3), 319-340 DOI: 10.1037//0033-295X.94.3.319

[11] http://berkeleysciencereview.com/can-mindfulness-make-you-happier/

[12] Miller, William R., and Stephen Rollnick. Motivational Interviewing: Helping People Change 3rd edition. New York: Guilford, 2013. Print.

[13] Move toward the goal. There is no assumption that we are actually free of judgment. Oh my gosh! Wouldn't that be great to achieve, but we mere humans simply need to focus on effort and progress, not the divine goal of perfection.

[14] This may be the greatest understatement in this whole manual.

[15] http://www.dictionary.com/browse/evocation

[16] Kabat-Zinn, Jon. "Wherever You Go, There You Are: Mindfulness Meditation in Everyday Life." New York: Hyperion, 1994. Print.

[17] Davis, Daphne, and Stephen Hayes. "What Are the Benefits of Mindfulness?" APA (2007): n. pag. Http://www.apa.org. APA. Web. 19 Sept. 2015. <http://www.apa.org/education/ce/ mindfulness-benefits.pdf

[18] "The Center for Mindful Eating - Good-Practice Guidelines." The Center for Mindful Eating - Good-Practice Guidelines. N.p., n.d. Web. 06 Feb. 2017.

[19] Kronick, Richard, Phd, Stephanie Chang, MD MPH, Jean Sultsky, PA MSPH, and Shilpa H. Amin, MD MBsc FAAFP. "Meditation Programs for Psychological Stress and Well-Being,"Agency for Healthcare Research and Quality 124 (2014): 1-143. Web.

[20] Eberth, Juliane, and Peter Sedlmeier. "The Effects of Mindfulness Meditation: A Meta-Analysis." Mindfulness 3.3 (2012): 174-89. Web.

[21] Sedlmeier, Peter, Juliane Eberth, Marcus Schwarz, Doreen Zimmermann, Frederik Haarig, Sonia Jaeger, and Sonja Kunze. "The Psychological Effects of Meditation: A Meta-analysis." Psychological Bulletin 138.6 (2012): 1139-171. Web.

[22] ibid Eberth, Juliane, and Peter Sedlmeier. "The Effects of Mindfulness Meditation: A Meta-Analysis." Mindfulness 3.3 (2012): 174-89. Web.

[23] Self-Compassion: The Proven Power of Being Kind to Yourself Kristin Neff - William Morrow & Company - 2015

[24] Siegel, Daniel J. *Mindsight: The New Science of Personal Transformation*. New York: Bantam Trade Paperbacks, 2011. Print.

[25] From HAESCommunity.Org, adapted from Body Respect: What Conventional Health Books Leave out, Get Wrong and Just Plain Fail to Understand about Weight, by Linda Bacon, PhD. and Lucy Aphramor, PhD, RD.

[26] "The Center for Mindful Eating - Principles of Mindful Eating." The Center for Mindful Eating - Principles of Mindful Eating. N.p., n.d. Web. 06 Feb. 2017.

[27] Bays, Jan Chozen., and Jon Kabat-Zinn. Mindful Eating: A Guide to Rediscovering a Healthy and Joyful Relationship with Food. Boston: Shambhala, 2009. Print.

[28] Albers, Susan. 50 Ways to Soothe Yourself without Food. Strawberry Hills, NSW: ReadHowYouWant, 2016. Print.

[29] Wansink, Brian. Mindless Eating: Why We Eat More than We Think. London: Hay House, 2011. Print.

[30] Golden, Nelville, Maria Schinder, and Christine Wood. "AAP Clinical Report : Steps to Prevent Teen Obesity and Eating Disorders." The American Academy of Pediatrics, 22 Aug. 2016. Web.

[31] The Tree of Contemplative Practices http://www.contemplativemind.org/practices/tree

[32] Siegel, Daniel J. "Attachment." Pocket Guide to Interpersonal Neurobiology: An Integrative Handbook of the Mind. New York: W.W. Norton, 2012. 20-8. Print.

[33] Brown, Brené. Rising Strong: The Reckoning. The Rumble. The Revolution. New York: Spiegel & Grau, 2015. Print.

[34] "Food for Thought Handout Archive 2006-2013." Issuu. The Center for Mindful Eating, n.d. Web. 06 Feb. 2017.

[35] Brown, Brené. Connections Curriculum A 12 Session Psycho-educational Shame Resilience Curriculum. N.p.: Hazen, 2009. Print.

[36] Brown, Brenè. "The Gifts of Imperfection." Center City: Hazelden, 2010. 46. Print.

[37] I placed "simply" in quotes because it is anything but simple.

[38] "Countertransference." MerriamWebster, n.d. Web.

[39] "The Healthy Mind Platter." Dr. Dan Siegel - Resources - Healthy Mind Platter. N.p., n.d. Web. 06 Feb. 2017.

[40] Four skills of Nonviolent Communication, https://www.cnvc.org/Training/NVC-Concepts

[41] NVC Feelings when satisfied, https://www.cnvc.org/Training/feelings-inventory

[42] "Right Intention: Samma Sankappa." Right Intention: Samma Sankappa. N.p., n.d. Web. 06 Feb. 2017.

[43] Webvague. "BJ Fogg's Motivation Wave." YouTube. YouTube, 30 May 2016. Web. 06 Feb. 2017.

[44] In Buddhist Teachings, Greed, Hatred, And Delusion Are Known, For Good Reason, As. "The Three Poisons." Transformingthethreepoisons : Greed, Hatred and Delusion(n.d.): n. pag. PrisonMindfulness.org. Web.

[45] "Amartya Sen." Wikipedia. Wikimedia Foundation, n.d. Web. 06 Feb. 2017. <https://en.wikipedia.org/wiki/Amartya_Sen>.

[46] Scientific Report of the 2015 USDA Dietary Guidelines Advisory Committee Part D. Chapter 5: Food Sustainability and Safety https://health.gov/dietaryguidelines/2015-scientific-report/10-chapter-5/

[47] "Definition of Ethics." Oxford Dictionaries. N.p., n.d. Web. <https://en.oxforddictionaries.com/definition/ethics>.

[48] The Tree of Contemplative Practices http://www.contemplativemind.org/practices/tree

Learn more about mindful eating from Megrette's other books:

BEST SELLER DISCOVER MINDFUL EATING

This book will give you the skills to use mindful eating in your practice! It's designed to give RDs and CDEs the practical tools to use mindful eating for weight loss, diabetes management, and disordered and emotional eating.

DISCOVER MINDFUL EATING FOR KIDS!

Ideal for Healthcare Professionals, Child Care Professionals, WIC Nutritionist who want to gain the skills and confidence to use mindful eating with the pint-sized set in your practice! Here are practical tools to use mindful eating for pediatric clients (and their parents) with a variety of challenges: picky eating, disordered and emotional eating, weight loss, and just to develop healthy and healthful eating habits.

Praise for this book from other professionals

"Great book! I enjoyed all the hands-on activities the book included. Since the book is geared towards children, the visuals really help drive the message home. I really enjoyed and learned so much from this book. I look forward to using everything I learned." — SHERVIN SOLIMANIJAN, RD, LOS ANGELES, CA

"The best part of these activities are the interaction with the child. It's an opportunity for the child to take part in the education, rather than just the parent." — CHRISTINA HOLMES, RD, LD, JOPLIN, MO

"These activities introduced new concepts to help kids think beyond eating food to fill them up. I like using these tools as part of my discussion about awareness of eating, hunger, fullness, and mindfulness with kids. It is nice to have activities to help them think and participate!" — SARA KUYKENDALL, MBA, RD, LD, WINCHESTER, VA

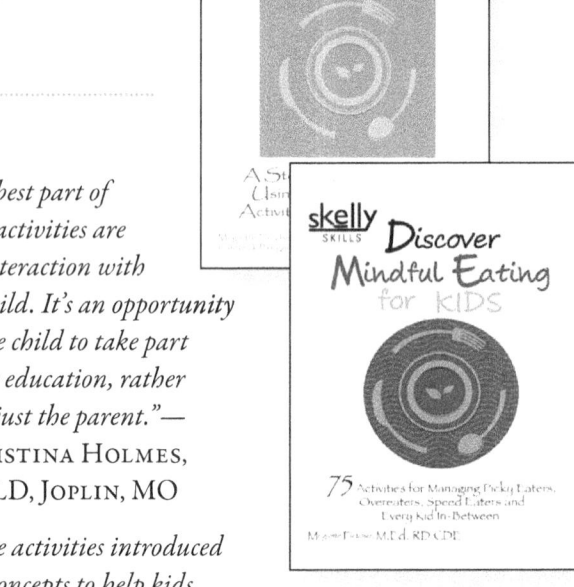

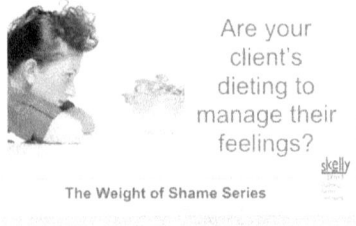

Enjoy Megrette's recorded webinars available at Skelly Skills and The Center for Mindful Eating, such as: The Weight of Shame: Understanding the importance of shame on your weight management clients.

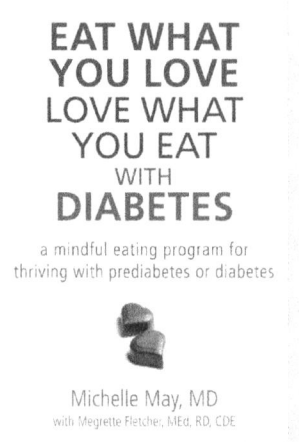

In depth Training Programs for professionals and their clients on how Mindful Eating can improve blood glucose control. Based on the Eat What You Love, Love What You Eat with Diabetes book, these programs are available at AmIHungry.com

Praise for the 3-Steps to Mindful Eating Bi-Annual Weekend Retreat

This retreat was an amazing way to deepen my already established mindful eating practice, and I believe it would be equally valuable for anyone from beginners to professionals. Megrette has a wonderfully unique way of meeting each participant where they're at and helping them to get the most out of the experience. I particularly enjoyed the intimate group size and the balance of both active and reflective techniques. The safe and supportive community that we established allowed for open sharing and lots of deep healing to take place. I left the retreat with a feeling of freedom and lightness along with lots of new techniques that I will use in my own practice in addition to sharing with others. I highly recommend this retreat to anyone who is looking to start or continue on a journey of eating mindfully, or who wishes to help others do the same. I will certainly be returning for the next retreat! — Traci, participant

"*The weekend retreat was such a welcoming experience. I have been able to integrate the mindfulness practice into so many areas of my life much more easily since the retreat. Each of you contributed in so many ways and for that I am grateful!*" — Kim, participant

"*I really loved the workshop. I got so much out of it.*" — Judy, participant

"*As a dietitian and CDE, I wholeheartedly recommend this workshop. It amplified my understanding of Mindful Eating concepts and gave me practical tools to use with my patients.*"— Caitlin Troklus, MS, RD, CDE

"*I left with clear guidance and many tools to use in my professional work as an RD in diabetes education..*" — Marianne Evans-Ramsay, RD, CDE

Praise for Megrette's Webinar Programs

"*I find it challenging in working with Motivational Interviewing to maintain a relational style and still focus on the process of MI. It was great to hear Megrette and "Kim" role play the process.*" — Julie, Webinar Participants regarding how to Professional working in diabetes benefit from using Mindful Eating.

"*I think this practical application of materials is very beneficial.*" — Webinar Participant regarding working with Shame

I serve as a preceptor for dietetic interns and listened with one of them yesterday. I found your analogy of Mindful Eating as a seed and Meditation, Self-Kindness and Non-Judgment as the roots a fascinating example! I also found it useful to imagine being judged, and "being" the judge — Lori Webinar Participants regarding 3-Roots of Mindful Eating

"*I appreciate the depth and breadth of your offerings. Lots of food for thought presented concisely and clearly. It has helped me improve my work with clients and my own struggle around mindful eating.*" — Webinar Participant regarding working with Shame

www.ingramcontent.com/pod-product-compliance
Lightning Source LLC
Chambersburg PA
CBHW081421230426
43668CB00016B/2308